# LIVIN' ON A CHAIR

## Lessons of Love, Work, and Faith

### after Breaking My Neck

# LIVIN' ON A CHAIR

## Lessons of Love, Work, and Faith

### after Breaking My Neck

*Jeff,*
*Hey man..! Enjoy the*
*story!*

# Scott Allen Frost

*PJH Publishing*

Cover art by George Wilson IV

Editing and layout Jonathan Peters, PhD

# THE SOUND

It's three seconds I relive everyday, several times a day...

I'm on a dirt bike. It's a perfect Southern Nevada day. Sun, blue sky, no humidity at 80 degrees.

I lay off the accelerator, pausing at the top of a concrete embankment, ready to catch my breath.

I feel my weight shift. Slightly off-balance. I look down to my right as my front tire begins slipping off the top of the wall.

My heart stops. It's a four foot drop. I know I'm going to hit hard, but I've had worse falls.

My left leg is still on the ground. Right foot still on the peg. I make a choice, the wrong choice, stay on the bike as it goes over.

I hold on hard to the handlebars, bracing for impact as the motorcycle turns perpendicular. My center of gravity is pulling me over the handlebars. I'm going down, straight down. I don't

1

have time to adjust before my head hits square on the crown of my head.

I'm shocked by the violence of the impact. I hear a loud CRACK. My body jolts with the power of it before slumping with the bike, flopping me on my stomach.

I relive those three seconds over and over. The shift in weight, the split-second decision, the falling, the sound, the physical jolt as all my weight pushes downward. And then the awkward angle in which I land.

And then the questions; "What if..." What if I'd just simply jumped off the bike? Or let go of handlebars? Put out my arms? Stuck out my leg? Tucked my head? What if I had ignored Cort's phone call. Gone to the movies with my kids?

And then I hear the sound. The shuttering, gut-wrenching sound.

# CHAPTER 1

# The Accident

It was Mother's Day, 2009. The morning started with me climbing out of my sleeping bag as the sun rose above the mountains surrounding Lake Mead. My kids and I were camping. We had spent the last few days playing in the water and hiking. In the evenings, we played horseshoes and poker late into the night under a full moon.

Which meant there wasn't much time relaxing Sunday morning. With the first rays of sunlight, I began breaking camp, while my kids, being teenagers, took their time waking up and moving around. I prodded them, making sure we got home in time to clean up before the kids spent the evening with their mother.

Finally, we had the SUV packed and were headed back to Las Vegas. When we got home, everyone rushed to unpack and clean up. While I was thinking about Mother's Day, I called my mom. I was looking down at the papers on my desk when my call went to voice mail. Distracted by all that I had to do, I accidently wished her a Happy Birthday instead of Mother's Day.

By this point, my children were back downstairs. My daughter, Taylor, teased me about my mistake. Then she and her younger brother, Christian, began reliving the weekend as they waited for their mother to arrive. The plan was to go to the movies and enjoy a meal afterward.

Their mother, Heather, and I had divorced five years earlier. And while things were difficult leading up to the break-up and the first few years afterward, Heather and I were on good terms.

After I called Heather to confirm that she was coming to get the kids, I joked around with Christian and Taylor for a couple minutes before my attention turned back toward my desk.

In that moment, I transitioned from enjoying my kids into full work mode. Unfortunately, this wasn't the first time my kids had seen this transition in me. I must have had an awareness of the impact it had on them because I do have a memory of them going quiet as I began moving papers around. I might not have been consciously aware of their disappointment, but a part of me took note of the looks they exchanged as they patiently waited for their mother.

In my defense, I had been able to set aside the two important proposals for the days we were camping on Lake Mead. But now that I was home and the papers were in front of me, I was eager to get back to work.

My new company was dependent on getting those two bids. The first one, the one I was working on that Mother's Day, was for a $400 million resort in Chandler, Arizona that needed a nightclub. My company was one of two they were considering to set up and operate the nightclub.

The other project we were working toward was a new restaurant in the Mandalay Bay Resort and Casino. We had yet to secure a lease, but we had investors and a concept that was ready for Mandalay Bay's consideration.

I looked up from my desk when Heather pulled into the driveway. The kids were animated again, excited to tell their mother about the camping trip. I put down the papers and closed my laptop and joined everyone in the entryway.

"Dad, come to the movies with us," Taylor pleaded.

I shook my head, "Nah, I have work to do."

"But Dad," Christian pitched in, "It's Star Trek."

I hugged him. "No, I have to get this done."

"Daaad," Taylor tried again.

I just shook my head as I hugged her as well, guiding both of them to the door.

I stood in the shade of the portico outside my front door as they loaded into Heather's car. When they were backing out of the driveway, I waved goodbye. My mind was already back on the proposal.

An hour later, my phone rang. I looked at the screen. Normally, I would have let it go to voicemail, but I was making good progress. Seeing Cortney Smith's name on the screen, I smiled. As a fellow entrepreneurs, Cort and I had known each other for more than a year, sharing with each other the burdens and joys of owning and running our own businesses.

"Hey, man." I answered.

He said, "Dude, it's a beautiful day. Let's go for a ride."

I'd been bugging him for months to get back on a motorcycle. Dirt bikes had been an important part of my life as a teenager and into adulthood. But when my kids were born, I sold my last motorcycle. Now that they were teenagers and I was single again, I had a desire to get back on a bike and feel the thrill of racing across the dessert.

As a child, my mother didn't want me to have a motorcycle. She would always warn, "You'll break your neck on those things."

She definitely wasn't happy when my dad bought me my first motorcycle when I was 13. I can remember her frowning at my father, blaming him for future injuries she could anticipate.

I was thrilled with that first motorcycle. Every opportunity I had, I'd be in the desert, popping over jumps, spinning out in corners, tearing across the flats.

As I got older, I loved being able to explore the hidden spots in Nevada. So much of this beautiful state is not accessible by pavement.

But, with the responsibility of children coming, Heather had convinced me to set aside motorcycles. That was years ago. Maybe it was time to start enjoying motorcycles again.

Cort, being a motorcycle enthusiast, wanted me to get back into riding. He often takes people on extended motorcycle trips, sharing with them the joy of riding. I felt badly about turning him down in the past. Rationalizing that I needed a break from the proposal, and that a little time in nature would get my creative juices going again, I said, "I've got to wrap this proposal up. Give me an hour, and I will be over."

I paused, thinking what else might be on my schedule. "But I have got to get my haircut later today. It's been eight weeks, man. I don't think I've ever gone this long without a cut."

Cort chuckled, "That's okay. We can just ride for an hour or so."

I was excited as I finished my thoughts, saved the documents, and sent out the final emails. I ran upstairs, put on some jeans and a long-sleeve shirt. Yes, I was a little nervous. I hadn't been on a bike in a while, but I was counting on what they say about riding a bicycle.

My Cadillac Escalade was one of the few luxuries I'd allowed myself after the divorce. And I hadn't settled for just any Escalade; this one had an amazing sound system because I love my rock and roll, and I like to play it loud.

I waited until I was out of my neighborhood, rolled down the windows and cranked the volume. I loved driving that truck, sitting up high, feeling the engine pull me through the curves. And pounding out the beats.

I'm a drummer, so as I drove, I tapped my foot like a kick drum, and pounded the steering wheel and dash like I was working the rest of the drum kit. And I sang at full volume with Kid Rock on *Cowboy*, and Green Day on *American Idiot*.

I'm a work hard/play hard guy. My work was done, and now I was rocking on my way to getting dirty in the desert. I felt excited, ready to take on the world.

When I got to Cort's, I jumped out, hugged him. I turned back to the Escalade, considering leaving my wallet and phone locked inside, but then thought better of it. Instead, I placed them in a pack with some water for the ride.

Cort and I chatted as we moved around the garage. He offered me a XR250 Yamaha, which was well within my range. I had ridden 500s before, so I knew I could easily handle the bike.

He rolled it into the driveway for me, and returned to the garage to get his bike. The problem was I hadn't kick-started a motorcycle in years. It took me a couple of tries before I got the engine going. Then I struggled with my helmet because I'd already put on my riding gloves. I considered leaving the strap loose, like I often did as a young man, but thought better of it. I took off the gloves, tightened the helmet strap, and put them back on.

Cort, of course, was set and ready to go, revving his engine while he waited for me to complete my preparations. Finally, I had everything in place. I looked over at him and gave him a thumbs up with a big grin.

He smiled back, pulled in his clutch, put his bike in gear, and pulled out in front of me. I did the same, feeling the click of the transmission beneath me. I let out the clutch slowly, letting the engine whine as it engaged. The bike pulled me forward, quickly falling in behind Cort.

We headed up the street. It was a gorgeous Las Vegas spring day. Not a cloud in the sky. No wind. Temperatures in the 80s. We couldn't ask for a better day to ride.

We threaded through his neighborhood to where the houses gave way to the desert. At the end of the road, they'd piled up boulders to keep people on the pavement. For Cort, it was easy to ride over the top of the rocks, but for me, it was a little bit scary. I couldn't get the gears right, and stalled the bike a couple of times. Then I couldn't get the bike started again because of the precariousness of being on a boulder. Eventually, Cort had to start my bike for me and help me through the boulders.

Finally, we were through and the desert lay in front of us. Cort opened it up and blew out across the open land.

I watched him go, and thought, "I'm going to kill myself if I try to keep up with him." So I backed off a bit as I went down the dirt road. When I bumped over some rocks, the adrenaline started going. I almost wrecked a couple of times trying to get a feel for the bike. But I was determined to get it.

Cort looked back and realized I was struggling. He circled back to me to give me some encouragement. Then he rode off for a bit before circling back again. Each time he got back to me, he'd give me a thumbs-ups or a high-five when I got through a tough spot. "You're doing great," he'd yell over the engines.

Eventually, we got to a huge water retention basin. It's a concrete area as big as a football stadium that holds water when it floods in Southern Nevada. The banks are around 40 feet high, sloping at 25 degrees.

They don't want people in the retention basin, so they stack big rocks all around the rim, maybe eight yards of rocks. By this time, I was getting a feel for the bike. I made it through the boulder field a little more easily, even though I'm sure I looked pretty awkward wobbling over one rock, trying to get to the next one, all while keeping my balance as I navigated through the obstacles.

Once inside the retention area, though, I started having fun. I could race across the concrete floor and zip up and down the embankments. We had lots of room to play, and without rocks and the uneven terrain of the desert, I felt more comfortable on the bike. My abilities were starting to come back. I was getting more and more daring.

On the embankments, there were these little abutments that jutted out. I'm not sure what they were for, but they made nice little jump ramps. I looked at one, braced myself, and went for it. Cort was watching as I landed it. He rode over, "Wow, man, I can't believe you did that."

I smiled and jumped twice more. Then I paused. I was getting out of breath and had to admit that I was a little tired. I decided I would ride to the top of an embankment and let the sweat dry while I watched Cort for a bit.

Cort knew where I was headed, so he chased after me, to wave me off. He knew this embankment dropped off on the other side. But I didn't see him waving me off. I was concentrating too much on maneuvering the motorcycle.

When I got to the top, it didn't flatten out like I'd expected. Instead, the top was rounded. And the other side dropped straight off for about four feet.

Instinctively, I put on my front brake, trying to keep on top. Seeing Cort, and noting what he was warning me about, I looked over. At that moment, with my balance shifting a bit, my front tire slowly slipped over the edge.

I knew the bike was going over. My instinct was to try to land it, to stay on the bike and follow through like I'd done on the jumps.

So I gripped the handlebars and prepared for the trip over the top. I knew I was going to crash, but I expected there to be enough momentum to carry me forward. I assumed the front tire would hit first and then I'd wipe out.

Four feet, no big deal. It wouldn't be my first crash of the day, and certainly not the first four-foot crash in my lifetime. It wasn't like I was going off a cliff or traveling 70 miles an hour. If I could just get the front tire up and maybe shoulder roll...

What I didn't anticipate was that by going so slowly over the edge, the bike turned perpendicular to the ground. But I'd already committed to riding out the fall. And now my head was ahead of the bike. My body was above me. I was confused by how the fall was playing out.

And then the sound, the shattering sound. A sound I can't describe, and that I can't erase. I hear it over and over, several times a day. It still haunts me.

# CHAPTER 2

# Paralyzed

I lay on my stomach, not knocked out, just stunned. And I was acutely aware that I couldn't move. This was bad, very bad.

My bike had done a perfect flip, and it was now on my back. The seat was on my shoulders and the handlebars rested across the back of my knees. It was still running.

My head had turned to the right, pressing my left ear into the ground. I could see my right arm resting six inches in front of my face.

And my left arm was trapped under my body from following the handlebars. From past football injuries, I knew that my left shoulder was dislocated. And now I was lying on it, unable to move off of it.

The pain was excruciating. And I was powerless to relieve it.

Cort saw the whole thing. He would have laughed at the sight of me lying there with the bike on my back, except I wasn't moving. He assumed I'd been knocked out, so he rushed to me.

He grabbed the bike off my back and turned it off. Seeing I was conscious he said, "Man, you hit your head pretty hard. Are you OK?"

It was then that I realized that I couldn't breathe. Even with the motorcycle off my back, I still felt like a huge weight was pressing down on me. I couldn't take in a deep breath. Something was wrong with my diaphragm.

In that moment, it dawned on me; I'd broken my neck.

Even though I couldn't feel below my chest, the pain in my shoulder was intense, I was aware of little else.

When the pain became overwhelming, I closed my eyes. Immediately, I got the sensation that I was floating in warm water. My arms felt like they were across my chest, and my knees were pulled up in the fetal position. It was a peaceful, calming sensation. My conscious brain knew I wasn't in the fetal position, even though it felt like some type of primitive return to the womb.

Panic forced my eyes open.

My first thoughts were that my mother was right. I did break my neck riding a motorcycle after all. It just took me 30 years. Here I was, on Mother's Day, paralyzed in a ditch in the middle of the desert.

I'd really done it. I had really messed up. And now I was scared.

"Cort, I've broken my neck. I can't move. I've broken my neck."

His demeanor immediately changed. Before, he was waiting for me to groan and roll over, so he could tease me about the fall. But now he knew I was in trouble.

I said, "You've got to get help. You've got to get help." Panic started to set in. What was I going to do?

Cort reached into his pack for his phone. Thank God we had a signal. Relief flooded through me when I heard those words, "911. What's your emergency."

I could endure the pain now that they'd be sending a helicopter to get me to the hospital. I knew I needed to get there quickly if there was any chance of me surviving. And now Cort had them on the phone, it'd be a matter of minutes.

Cort was calm and serious. Of course he was scared, but he kept his head. He told the 911 operator where we were, which was harder than you might think. We were in the middle of the desert in an undeveloped canyon, down in a flood retention basin. If you were standing 100 yards away in any direction, you couldn't see us or the basin we were in. There was no rock out-cropping, power line, tree, or anything. Just desert.

Cort knew we were in Madera Canyon. He said, "We are in the flood retention basin, approximately five miles south of the Henderson airport. We have a rider with a broken neck. We need a Life Flight.

She kept asking, "What are the cross streets?"

"No cross streets. We're in Madera Canyon, in a flood reten-tion basin. We need a Life Flight."

I remember being frustrated because she kept asking for cross streets and Cort kept repeating his information. "You don't understand. We are not in a suburban area. We aren't on any streets. We are out in the desert. Five miles south of the Henderson Airport. When you get a flight up, they'll be able to see us."

Cort did his best to keep his frustration under check, but I began to get mad. Why couldn't she understand? Just get a chopper up and find me.

Then things got worse. The operator explained that they couldn't simply send out a helicopter for us. First, a terrestrial-based search-and-rescue team must confirm the severity of the injury. Only they could call in a helicopter. This was in 2009, and the City of Henderson wanted to make sure I didn't just have a broken leg before spending the money on a helicopter. If my accident had occurred anywhere else in the Las Vegas valley, Metro would have sent a Life Flight right away. But this was Henderson.

Also, in 2009, we didn't have GPS on our phones, so Cort had no way to lead the Fire and Rescue department to us.

Cort went back and forth with the operator, trying to paint a picture of where we were. More than 20 minutes went by before we heard sirens, but they sounded miles away.

Now Cort had a dilemma; does he leave me and ride out to the nearest paved road, which was probably two miles away, and flag one of these guys down? What would happen if they didn't find him? What would happen to me?

I said, "Cort, light one of the motorcycles on fire, and they will see the smoke."

He seriously considered it, saying "I'm not going to leave you."

The truth was I didn't want to be left alone. It was becoming increasingly difficult for me to breathe. As time passed, it became difficult to speak. I could only mumble a couple of sentences, gasping every four or five words.

The pain from my shoulder became more intense. It was the worse pain I'd ever had, and I was still lying on the shoulder 20 minutes after the accident. And the pavement was hot.

Oddly, my neck didn't hurt, even though I knew it was broken. There was also a serious cut on my shin that I couldn't feel. And evidently my nose was broken from where the helmet had pushed down on the bridge.

And I knew I had a concussion.

But none of that was bothering me. My adrenaline was pumping, so I was clear headed. I knew what the circumstances were and what was going on. Which meant that I was very aware that I couldn't move, that the concrete was hot, that all I could see was my right hand and the wall I'd fallen from, that my life would never be the same, and there was nothing I could do to help myself.

"I don't want to die." I told Cort.

"Don't worry, Buddy, we're going to take care of you. We're going to get you out of here."

"I don't want to die." I repeated.

Cort looked over, "No one is going to die today, Buddy. We're getting you out of here."

# CHAPTER 3

# Glimmer of Hope

Just when it began to look like Fire and Rescue would never find us, Cort saw a mountain biker a long way off.

How loud would you yell to save someone's life? Cort yelled louder than that. It was blood curdling. He screamed, "Help Me! Hey! Hey! Hey! Help Us! Oooover hereeee!" Cort jumped up and down, waving his arms.

Cort got the guy's attention. He turned his bike toward us. It wasn't any easier for him to get over the rocks around the edge of the basin, so he dropped his bike and ran until he was close enough to hear what Cort was saying, "My friend has broken his neck. Those sirens you hear, they are looking for us. But they don't know how to get to us."

The bike-rider said "I know where to go." He ran back to his bike and took off.

Now, at least, we knew someone was out there to flag down one of the sirens. Cort described the man to the 911 operator,

"He's wearing a white T-shirt, black riding shorts. He's on a mountain bike. Look for this guy. He will guide you in."

"What's he driving."

"He is on a mountain bike."

Now that we had hope, my mind began to wander. I'd been around a lot of quadriplegics and paraplegics in the past, so I knew what I was in for. I spent the first six years of my career in pharmaceutical sales. One of my accounts was a leading spine injury hospital at Stanford. Since paralyzed people have a lot of urinary track infections and trouble sleeping, I sold the hospital antibiotics and sleep agents. From working with doctors at the hospital, and meeting with different patients, I knew what type of life I was I was facing.

Now that my fear was reducing, anger began to rise up. The more I thought about my new reality, the more angry I became.

I could be watching *Star Trek* with my kids instead of lying in a ditch in the middle of nowhere. I would forever be a burden on my family. My parents were in their 70s; they couldn't take care of me. Worse than the physical burden, what about the financial burden? No parent should have to take care of their adult child. I knew my mom and dad would be heart broken.

And my children were still young. What would their life be like? I was 6'7" and 280 pounds at the time of the accident. I was a big man who loved to hug. I'd pick up my children and spin them around. I was active with them, always playing. My kids' lives would never be the same. They'd have a cripple for a father.

Then I thought about my business. What would happen to my business? How would I support my family?

While I lay on the hot concrete, staring at my hand and the wall, I reviewed who I knew who had run a successful business without the use of their arms and legs. Christopher Reeves, certainly, but then I remembered reading an article about Ameristar CEO, Craig Neilson, who was a quadriplegic from a car accident. He literally ran his casino empire from his bed. I would simply need to find someone who knew Craig Neilson, and who could tell me exactly how he did it.

16

All this was going through my head, and I still couldn't move. My left arm was still stuck underneath my body. The pain in my shoulder was immense, and I couldn't feel anything else from my chest down.

And the minutes continued to pass.

Cort used my phone to call a friend of his who worked for a helicopter company nearby. He thought maybe his friend could circumvent the bureaucracy and get a chopper in the air. But his friend wasn't answering his phone.

Cort looked over at me, "Stay with me, Buddy."

I was becoming less responsive. I started to drift out of consciousness. As I struggled for breath, I realized that I might die before Fire and Rescue got to us. So I concentrated on my family and everything I wanted to do in life. I was scared, and sad; this might be the time and place where the Scott Frost story ends.

"I don't want to die." I repeated.

"No one is dying today, Scott. We're going to get you out of here."

I imagined the little blurb in the paper, "Henderson man died of a broken neck on Mother's Day... Left behind two kids..." Faceless to those who read it. Anyone seeing the blurb would forget it minutes later.

That's when my phone rang. Cort looked at the caller ID; it was my mother. She was calling in reply to the mixed-up voice message I'd left her earlier, accidently wishing her a happy birthday.

Cort answered, "Gayle, this is Cort. There's been an accident. I'm with Scott. He's broken his neck."

She gasped, "Do we need to come down to Las Vegas?"

"Yes. You need to come. It's serious," Cort said. "I'll call you back as soon as I know more."

She said, "You take care of him. You take care of him."

"I will."

I could hear their conversation. Again, guilt, and the sorrow of burdening my parents, washed over me. For the first time, I began to cry. I could only imagine what my mother was going through with my dad. It was gut wrenching.

Just then a Henderson police officer in a Suburban pulled up to the rocks surrounding the retention area. He jogged the hundred yards to where we were.

"Thank God, I'm still alive," I thought.

I asked, "Officer, do you have GPS or longitude/latitude that gives us a 20 as to where we are? Can you give it to the Fire Department?"

He replied, "I can't talk to them; we don't have a direct line to Fire. We are going to have to talk through the 911 dispatch."

I was dumbfounded. My heart sank. Worse, he didn't have an electronic method of pinpointing our location. All he could do was what Cort had been doing, talk to 911 dispatch. And she still wasn't understanding where we were and what the situation was.

The only directions we could give were, "Go to the end of this street, take a right, hit a dirt road, head approximately a quarter of a mile, and then bear left..." Now, though, we had a landmark—his big, white suburban in the middle of nowhere.

Finally, the sirens got louder, and I asked, "Is Life Flight on the way?"

"No. Search and Rescue has to see you first," the officer said.

I cursed. I couldn't believe he couldn't call a helicopter. It was obvious I need one.

While we waited, the man on the mountain bike returned. To this day, I don't know his name. Without him, who knows if the cop would have ever found us. And I'm certain Fire and Rescue would have never reached me before I died. I hope to someday be able to thank the man on the mountain bike. If you know him, or are him, please get in touch with me.

Now that the sirens were approaching, I started to do the math in my head. *We were 35 minutes into the crisis. It's going to take Fire and Rescue another 30 to find me and get a helicopter to me. There's no way I'm going to last. I'm running out of air.*

The officer knelt down next to me and patted my shoulder. "Hang in there."

# CHAPTER 4

# Saying Goodbye

When I realized that I probably wouldn't make it, I thought of all the people I would be leaving behind: my parents, my family, my friends, my girlfriend Megan, but most of all my children.

Imagine having the opportunity to know you're about to die, and to be able reach out to your loved ones in the final moments. Few people have this opportunity. Usually death surprises us. But in my case, I still had time.

I didn't want my kids to hear about my last moments from someone else. I didn't want them wondering what my last thoughts were. Was I thinking of them when I passed? Was I afraid? I needed to talk to them now.

"Cort, call Heather. She is in a movie with the kids. Keep calling until she picks up."

He said, "Scott, are you sure you want me to do this?"

"Yes."

He dialed, but of course she didn't answer. Cort called again. Then again. Now she would know something was wrong.

The movie was just ending as Cort was calling. Taylor ran to the restroom with her friend CJ who had joined them for the movie. Christian and Heather waited in the lobby.

Heather answered this time, "Hello, Scott."

"It's Cort. Scott's been in an accident."

Christian saw the look on his mother's face. "What?"

Heather asked, "How bad is it?"

"Bad, very bad. He's broken his neck and is losing consciousness."

Christian was becoming hysterical. "What? What?"

Distracted, Heather said, "Your father's been in an accident, and it's serious. He might not make it."

Reacting to his mother's expression and words, Christian lost it. Right there in the lobby of the theater, in front of the concession stands, my 14-year-old son fell to the floor and began wailing.

That's what Taylor and CJ saw when they came back from the restroom. "What's happened?"

"Your father has been in an accident."

"Is he okay?"

"No."

That one word told Taylor more than she wanted to know. She didn't know that I was dirt biking that afternoon. She thought I was simply in a car accident. And of course my big SUV would protect me.

Heather motioned for the kids to follow her out of the theater. The theater they'd chosen for the movie is in a casino. So they had a long walk to the parking garage. The whole way, Heather peppered Cort with questions, trying to get a better understanding of my situation.

The kids were too distraught to understand what was going on. Plus, they were only hearing Heather's side of the conversation.

Finally, they reached their car and got in. Christian continued to scream, Taylor tried to comfort him while Heather asked to talk to me.

Cort put the phone on speaker mode and laid it on the ground next to my face.

"I'm sorry," I said.

Heather, said, "Scott, I love you. Hang in there."

I said, "Let me talk to the kids."

She handed the phone to Taylor. What do you say to your kids if you have one minute to say good-bye for the last time? I could hear my son screaming.

I began to sob. "I love you so much. I love you so much. I'm so sorry. Be good. I love you so much. I'm sorry."

Taylor didn't understand the situation. She didn't understand that this was good-bye. She certainly didn't understand what I was sorry about. "It's going to be okay. Daddy Man can't go," she said, referring to an old joke of ours.

"Take care of each other," I said.

"Yes, Dad. Do you want to speak with Christian?"

"Yes."

She handed the phone to Christian who just screamed into the phone. I couldn't comfort him. I couldn't be the strong father who was always there to pick him up and wrap him in my arms. All I could repeat was, "I'm sorry. I love you," as I started to drift into despair.

The officer picked up the phone from the ground. "You need to keep him talking. We are losing him. You have to keep him talking."

Heather took back the phone. "Scott, you've got to hang in there. Talk to me."

Heather began to ask me if I remembered certain times with the kids, Christmas, movies we'd seen, trips we had taken.

The officer patted my back as I responded to Heather. When I started apologizing to Heather again, the officer asked me, "Where'd you grow up?"

"Reno."

He asked me other biographical questions to keep me talking.

I was losing energy. I couldn't talk any more. Their voices became distant, almost like they were in another room talking through a wall.

I am a man of faith. I was raised in the Lutheran church and was baptized as an infant. I had an on-and-off relationship with God. When I needed Him, He was always there. But when times were good, I tended to forget Him. I was a once-a-month church-goer. While I hadn't been praying much lately, I knew God was watching over me.

When the voices of Heather, my children, and the police officer faded, and I was still staring at that wall. I finally thought to pray, "Father, look over my kids. Take care of my kids. Bless my family. Keep them safe."

Then I said, "Please take me quickly. Please make it pain-less."

Just then the most amazing feeling washed over me, and a sense of calm and peace filled my body. All my pain and tension left. The only way I can describe it is, imagine every worry and every physical pain and all dissidence and worry disappears. What would you feel? It was complete peace.

In church, we'd said, "Peace be with you." This was the first time I understood the magnitude of "peace," at least in the way God meant it. It's the peace that passes understanding.

We've been in peaceful places, felt content, but there is nothing like the calm and peace that washed over me in that moment. This is the peace that is waiting for all of us. This is the peace that, if we had 100% faith, we could have on this earth.

I had the sensation of being cradled. Arms reached underneath my knees and my back. I closed my eyes, and my last conscious thought was, "I wonder what this is going to feel like." I had a sense of pure love enveloping me, filling my heart. Then the cradling arms began to lift me upward.

# CHAPTER 5

# In Flight

Suddenly, pounding noise was all around me. I squinted up at blue sky. I was being jostled, and people were moving in my peripheral vision.

As I regained consciousness, I realized I was no longer staring at a concrete wall. Instead, I had been flipped onto my back. The pounding noise was from a helicopter. I counted three people working on me. I could see an IV bag above me, and assumed a needle was in my arm. They'd cut my shirt off me. Looking down at my chest, I could see heart monitor suction cups taped to me. I could also tell that I was strapped to a spine board.

Cort later told me that from the time I stopped talking, to the time that the helicopter got there, was about four minutes. He considered rolling me over and giving me CPR. But he had the wherewithal to keep checking my pulse. He decided as long as I had a pulse, he'd leave me where I was. Fortunately, the helicopter got there before my heart gave out. Seconds more, who knows what might have happened.

What kept me alive was a small amount of oxygen remaining in my lungs. When I passed out, I wasn't expending any more energy, so I had just enough air to keep me alive until the rescue team arrived. A minute or two later, they would not have been able to bring me back.

The moment I realized that I was going to make it after all, I became elated. I was going to live! I was going to see my family again! I said aloud, within the cacophony of the spinning chopper blades, "This is not going to be the end of my story. This is the new beginning."

I don't know where I was getting this bravado, but I remember telling Cort. "Take pictures. This is going to be the comeback story of the year."

He had only moments to get a couple pictures before they were ready to get me out of the ditch and into the helicopter.

That's when they ran into a problem. At 6' 7", I don't fit nicely on a spine board. And then I had a helmet on, which made me even longer. My feet were hanging well off the board. When we got to the helicopter, they couldn't figure how to get me inside. They would put me in one way, try to wiggle me in, then remove me and try a different approach. After several tries they had me in just enough to be able to close the doors.

"Have you ridden in a helicopter?" one of the paramedics yelled at me.

"No."

"Be prepared. You might be nauseated."

With that, they swooped away, heading straight to the University Medical Center.

They asked me a bunch of questions, like, "What happened? How did you hurt yourself? Did you hear any cracks? Did you hear anything?"

I replied, "I hit my head really hard. I know I have a concussion..."

Then I paused. With all the attention on stabilizing my neck, no one had bothered to look at my shoulder. The pain was still intense. I asked the paramedic, "Can you do me a favor?"

He said, "What?"

"I know I've dislocated my shoulder, and I know you are worried about my spine, but my shoulder is really killing me."

He looked down, noticing my shoulder for the first time. He pulled on my arm and the socket slid into place. It was instant relief.

They then continued with the questions. I answered as best I could. Now that my shoulder wasn't hurting, I could focus. In less than fifteen minutes, I felt our momentum shift. Then we began to descend.

# CHAPTER 6

# Intake

When we landed at the hospital, a team of doctors was waiting. With spine injuries, time is of the essence. They needed to get a diagnosis quickly. Was the spine severed or contused? Is anything orthopedically putting pressure on the spine? They've got to get me on steroids immediately to bring down the swelling. All this will dictate how quickly I could go into surgery and ultimately my chances of recovery.

They cut off my pants and removed my shoes and socks. I was lying naked under a sheet, but I still had the big helmet on my head. It needed to come off before they could X-ray me.

They unbuckled the spine board and gingerly put a neck brace on me. Next, they transferred me to a gurney. I was scared because you always hear stories about people moving the neck the wrong way and their injury is made worse. Now they had to somehow get the helmet off my head without straining my neck. And it was on tight.

I felt two people get on either side of me. Another guy stood above me saying things like, "Stabilize him. Hold him. Ready?" But I couldn't see who was talking; I could only feel pressure as whatever slack there was between the helmet and my head was taken up.

"Ready?" the disembodied voice asked again. "Okay, One. Two. Three."

I could feel the pressure on my head as the helmet began sliding up. My ears twisted, until the helmet was passed them. Then suddenly I was free of the constriction. Not only did I have the pressure off my head, but I could now see more out of the corner of my eyes.

They wheeled me to the X-ray machine and began taking pictures. As soon as I could, I asked, "Is anything broken? Is my spine severed?"

No one would answer me. Instead, they said, "We've got to get you an MRI."

I tried again, "Will someone please tell me, is my spine severed?" All I wanted was the results from the X-ray.

But they said "We haven't seen your films. We've got to do a head-to-toe MRI to find out if you've broken any other bones or have any other injuries."

I knew from previous MRIs that I have a problem with claustrophobia. Being a big guy in a small tube is a sensation I don't like. "Can you give me some Valium before putting me in?"

"We already have you on morphine. Your breathing is compromised."

Another guy snapped at me, "Hey, if you don't want to do this right now. We can wait."

I interrupted, "Listen, asshole, if you want to trade places with me, go right ahead. I've broken my neck. My life is changed forever. I hate MRI machines."

I took a calming breath, "Just blindfold me. Is there any kind of music to distract me?"

Someone said, "We will blindfold you."

A cloth came over my eyes. But even in my state, I could still feel the enclosed space as they put me in the tube. And I remained there for nearly an hour. It was just me, alone with my thoughts. I couldn't move. It was absolute hell. I struggled with fits of panic, which were compounded by thoughts about my family, my kids, and the rest of my life.

As soon as I was out and could take a few breaths and relax, I pleaded, "Just someone tell me, did I sever my spine?"

Finally, someone said, "Your films are negative."

I wasn't used to not being able to see who was talking. My head was locked in place and everyone was moving around. I couldn't keep track of who was saying what. I called out, "Negative, as in nothing's broken?"

He said, "Negative. You did not break your vertebrae."

"So my spine is not severed?"

"It does not appear to be severed."

I knew enough to be relieved that my spine wasn't severed. That was good news. I shed a tear in relief. All was not lost. There was still a chance.

It would be months before I got the full diagnosis. By hitting the crown of my head, my head snapped straight back. I tore all the ligaments in the front part of my neck, and the spine itself was compressed. The disc between C3 and C4 was crushed and pushed forward. My paralysis was a function of two things: The spinal cord being compressed, and the disc pushing on the back part of my spine. The disc robbed my spine of oxygen, thus causing permanent damage.

But that day in the emergency room, I didn't know any of this. What I did know was that since I hadn't severed my spine, I had a glimmer of hope. If all I had were a contusion, I might be able to move someday.

I remembered the famous Buffalo Bills football player, Kevin Everett, who was paralyzed on national TV. They treated him with cold saline on the sidelines. The team owner was a big benefactor to a spine injury treatment facility, so they had an IV ready to go when Everett was injured.

It was a new treatment, but one that had received much study.

I knew that the number one thing that causes paralysis is swelling. Steroids are the usual approach to limiting swelling, but I wanted cold saline. I remember saying, "I need the cold saline. Get me the chilled saline. I want what that football player got."

When no one responded, I pushed it, "I want state-of-the-art. I want the best doctor in here. I want whatever it takes. Whatever it costs. I have great insurance."

The surgeon on duty looked at me and said, "That protocol has not been proven."

"But the football player ended up walking," I protested. "He walked onto the field the following season. "

The surgeon nodded and said, "The main course is steroids. We need to get the swelling down."

Then the assessments began. People kept touching and prodding while asking, "Can you feel this? Can you feel that? Can you grip this at all? Close your eyes. Can you feel this? Which leg am I touching. They were doing this on my arms, hands, torso, legs, and feet. I could feel a little bit on my right foot. I knew they were pressing something sharp into it. But my left foot felt nothing. My arms and hands were also numb.

I closed my eyes. All their questions were disheartening. I was trying, but I couldn't give them the answers I wanted to give.

Finally, they were done. They moved me to the ICU, and the surgeon came in to talk with me. He said, "When it comes to spinal cord injury, they are like snowflakes. No two snowflakes are the same. We have some general protocols like steroids to bring down the swelling, and surgery. After that, it's wait and see."

Cort was the first of my friends and family to come into my ICU room. With all the time I had to think in the MRI. I had a long list of things to unload on him. For instance, I told him to call my business partner, "Tell Jeff, don't stop. Move forward. I'll get the file emailed to him. The nightclub proposals is due Wednesday."

We'd put three years of our lives into getting this business off the ground. We'd taken money from investors and this was the gig that was finally going to pay some bills. All we had to do was push to the finish line.

While I was giving Cort directions, my ex-wife, Heather, came into the room. To give us a moment, Cort left the room to make phone calls.

Heather had tears in her eyes. She didn't say anything, just turned her iPhone toward me. On the screen was a picture of Jesus. I thanked her and closed my eyes. And then the tears came. I remembered the embrace I felt as I was dying in the desert. I was still alive because when I had given up, He hadn't given up on me.

Heather said, "We are praying for you. I left the kids with Rebecca (a family friend)."

I said, "I don't want the kids to see me like this. Do not bring them down here."

Heather nodded, understanding.

Cort came back with the phone. He put in on speaker and set it on the bed next to my head. Jeff, my partner, was shaken. "How bad is it?"

I knew he wanted to hear me say it wasn't bad, or that I'd be all right soon. All I could say was, "It's bad. It's serious."

I went on to tell him, "I did hit my head, but I had my helmet on, so I will be okay. I'm paralyzed, but from the shoulders up, I'm the same guy. All my mental facilities are with me. The only thing that has changed is the physical shell I'm in. We've got to finish that document and get it turned in Wednesday, and then we will go from there."

He started asking a bunch of questions, and I interrupted him, "Don't worry about me. They are going to take care of me. I'm going to be okay."

I assured him that most of what I do anyway is talk on the phone, and I can do that from a hospital bed. We needed to move forward as if nothing had happened.

We heard that my parents were on their way from Reno, and so was my brother from Phoenix.

In the meantime, the hospital staff was pumping me full of steroids to take the swelling down, and morphine to relax me and deal with the pain. It wasn't long before the adrenaline wore off and I began to fade.

Before I knew it, I was asleep.

# CHAPTER 7

# Megan

When I woke up hours later, it was dark and quiet. It took me a moment to orient myself. I strained my eyes left and then right attempting to get as much of a view of my surroundings as I could without moving my head.

I could sense that there was a person in the room. I couldn't move to see who it was, so I strained my eyes to the sides trying to see into the darkness. Perhaps I grunted or made some sound to alert them that I was now awake

The next thing I saw was Megan moving into my field of vision.

I can't describe the instant emotions I felt. Relief. Strength. Love. I hadn't seen her in two months, and I certainly didn't expect to see her at that moment.

My first thought was how beautiful she is. An angel in my room. I wanted to cry.

Megan and I met four and half years earlier, and had been together for years. She had become a part of my life and my kids' lives.

But a couple months before my accident, I messed up in a big way. We had spent the day off the coast of Laguna Beach with several friends. I was day drinking and was pretty well blasted as the party continued at my friend's house. In a drunken state, I did something incredibly stupid. The result was deeply hurting an amazing woman, the one who had helped me heal after my divorce, the woman who made me whole again.

When we returned to Las Vegas, Megan moved out of my house and wasn't speaking to me. My kids were distressed that she was no longer a part of our family and I didn't have the words to explain the situation to them.

It killed me to see my son withdrawing again. Just like after the divorce, Christian was spending most of his time in his room, not coming out, not talking.

I knew that I had not only hurt Megan, I'd also disrupted my children's lives. Once again, I was pursuing my own selfish desires, and my bad judgment, while under the influence, had cost me and hurt them. There were no excuses, and I totally understood Megan's position.

Which isn't to say that I didn't try to repair what I'd done and have Megan back in my life. I kept texting, calling, and emailing her in the weeks after she moved out.

I was a mess, an absolute mess. Classically heart-broken, I was despondent and depressed. I didn't want to get up in the morning and was listless at work.

I remember my daughter, Taylor, consoling me. "Dad, I know you'll end up together." She patted me on the leg. "I know she'll come back."

"I don't know..."

"Nah, it'll be okay. You two make a good couple."

A whole month passed without Megan in my life. My heart literally ached. We had been looking forward to attending a

Killers concert together, and now I was heading to it by myself. The whole time I was at the concert, I was thinking how much Megan would have enjoyed it. Finally, I texted, "I wish you were here."

She texted back, "I wish I was too."

The next day, we started talking on the phone. She said the reason she hadn't been answering my calls and texts was because she wanted to see if she'd miss me after moving out of my house. With all my haranguing, she hadn't had the opportunity to see if she'd miss me.

So it wasn't like Megan was totally out of my life when the accident happened. I simply didn't have faith that we'd end up back together.

Now, here she was, in my room, when I needed her the most, looking down on me from above.

I'll always remember the look on her face. It wasn't pity, nor anxiety, nor distress. She looked at me, and said, "We got this. I'm not going anywhere. We got this."

I started to cry. I couldn't believe that she had come back.

And come back she did, in a big way.

Megan hasn't left my side since. Imagine, you're young and you've broken up from this difficult man. You owe him nothing. You have a full life and amazing opportunities ahead of you. And yet, when I was in need, she came rushing back.

It was Taylor who called Megan.

Back at the parking garage, after police officer ended my call, Heather called CJ's mother, Rebecca, to pick up the kids so she could go to the hospital to be with me. But once Rebecca arrived and Heather left, no one knew what to do. Heather was gone. If the kids went to her house, that was all the way out in Boulder City. Meanwhile their mother was headed in the other direction to University Medical Center.

Rebecca asked, "Where do you want to go."

Taylor replied, "Church."

She wasn't active in the church yet, mostly because I wasn't. But at that moment, she knew she needed to pray.

Our church has a main sanctuary that seats 800, and a little chapel that seats 120. When they got to the church, Taylor rushed in, obviously distraught. She was looking down at her shoes when a man approached to help.

"Where can I pray?" she asked.

He guided her to the chapel, where she prayed for me for over an hour. It helped her get calm and collected so she could help her brother and face the hours and days ahead.

And that's when she thought to call Megan. Taylor was close to Megan, and instinctively knew Megan would not only want to know about my accident, but would also want to help. Taylor also knew that no one else would think to call Megan. So Taylor, in all her distress, reached out to the one person I needed the most.

Megan was at work when Taylor called, so she didn't answer the first few times. Eventually she picked up her phone, "Is everything okay?"

"No. Dad's been in an accident." Taylor told Megan that she didn't have any details and suggested Megan call Heather.

As soon as Megan could, she came to the hospital. By that time, everyone had left. It was as quiet as an ICU can be. Megan was the only visitor in the ward, but the nurses let her see me.

Megan knew there would be difficult times ahead. That she would be sacrificing much to be with me. Even though, at the time, we didn't know the extent of my injury, or how the rest of my life would turn out, she never questioned her decision. From that moment, she dedicated herself to me.

I would not, could not, be where I am today without Megan. And I don't just mean this in a romantic, sentimental way. When you're as helpless as I've been, you rely intensely on others. Everything I needed, she was there to take care of. If my face itches, she'd scratch it. If I needed water, she got it for me. Anything the nurses couldn't do for me, she did.

From that moment on, Megan spent every night with me. She wasn't supposed to be in the ICU after visiting hours, but most of the nurses realized how important it was that she be there, so they overlooked her presence.

There was one charge nurse who told Megan that she'd have to leave. The other nurses would watch for this nurse and tell us when she was headed our way. Megan would hide in the closet until we got the all-clear from the other nurses.

Because she wasn't supposed to be there, the nurses couldn't bring Megan a cot. So we improvised. Megan scooted a chair next to my bed, curled as best she could in the chair while draping her upper body on my bed, resting her head on my chest.

But the chair would not stay in place. As Megan's weight shifted in sleep, the chair would eventually squawk as it moved backward away from the bed. The noise would startle Megan, who'd jump awake, which of course startled me.

She'd carefully move the chair back into place, lay her head back down on me, and go back to sleep.

It seemed like I'd just be drifting back asleep when that chair would make that awful noise and wake us both up.

Sleep was illusive for me. After being awakened, I'd stare at the ceiling, listening to Megan breathing while I worried. In those long nights, it seemed like the chair made that noise a hundred times, keeping me in a wakeful state.

In the morning, Megan would clean up and get ready to head to work as soon as my parents showed up to relieve her.

I was so thankful to have her there. For some reason, I felt more paralyzed at night. There were fewer nurses around. It was quiet. I had more time to think. I would experiment throughout the night, trying to move my arms or a toe. And nothing would move. It was as if my body was encased in concrete.

Without Megan with me at night, I easily would have lost it. As irritating as it was, that sliding chair kept reminding me that I was loved and supported, and that, "We got this."

# CHAPTER 8

# "I Want to Live"

From the moment I was awake that first morning, people began streaming into my ICU room. My brother, Steve, had gotten in late the night before, so he was in my room the moment they let visitors in.

As soon as he walked in, my mind flashed back to a ski trip a few years earlier. We were sitting on the chairlift discussing an accident that had left someone paralyzed. I told Steve, "If that ever happens to me, it's your job to put a pillow over my face. I don't want to live like that."

When he walked into my ICU room that morning, our eyes locked, and I knew what he was thinking. I said aloud, "I want to live."

Before we had a chance to talk about it, more people began showing up. I couldn't believe how quickly word had traveled. And the phones in the room were ringing. Family and friends caught everyone up on what had happened.

Amidst all the activity, I dipped in and out consciousness. The trauma to my body, plus the medications, meant I didn't have the energy I would have liked for my visitors.

With so many people milling around, and hospital staff and medical professionals coming in and out of my room, we needed some way to keep track of everything. Megan created a system for keeping some sort of order to the chaos. We had a journal that was part diary, part organizing system. If you were in the room and you heard something, it was your responsibility to write it down.

University Medical Center is a teaching hospital, so residents kept coming by, poking and prodding. There would be a doctor teaching them, quizzing them about protocol, "What should we be looking out for..." It was fascinating. I learned right along with the residents.

Your modesty goes flying out the window when you're a quadriplegic. You literally can't do anything for yourself. You are going to be changed like a baby, fed like a baby, and poked and prodded and examined twice over.

I was blessed to have a network of people who cared about me. Very early on, I adopted the attitude that people don't like to help someone who doesn't want to help themselves. The worst thing I could do was to give up on myself. I needed to be cognizant that this was as hard on them as it was on me. If I broke down, they would break down. So I made a conscious effort to be upbeat for them.

For instance, one friend came to visit me. He walked in the room, saw me, turned, and walked back out. He apologized to Megan in the hall, "I can't stand to see him like that. I don't want to see him like that."

So I learned to brace myself for the reactions people would have, and then to reassure them that despite what I looked like, I was still the same old Scott Frost.

Like when Megan's parents came in. Her father, Johnny, didn't say anything. He stood there, looking at me. Then his lips started to quiver until he broke down crying. That was startling because Johnny is a former sailor; he still drinks and cusses like one. To witness how my situation affected him helped me see through other people's eyes.

I didn't realize how the visual of me, a big guy, laid out like that would shock people. In their minds they still saw the big hugger who'd wrestle them into a head lock. Now they're confronted with a shell of a man who can't even turn his head in greeting.

I said, "Johnny, come on, man. It's going to be OK. I'm still going to be able to kick your ass in poker. And I won't let you touch my chips."

He smiled through the tears and patted my shoulder.

Megan's mother showed me her Blackberry. On it was the last picture of me standing as my former self. It was taken as I was breaking down camp the day before at Lake Mead.

My former roommate, Jim, also came by. It didn't take him long to identify a problem for me. The television was on the wall, but with my head locked into place and I was flat on my back, my entire universe was a space of nine square feet of ceiling tiles above me.

Jim went home and got a projector. He set it up so I could watch movies on the ceiling. Since he knew my favorite movies, Jim also made sure I was well stocked with DVDs. It was one of the best gifts and gestures I received in those first few days. During the day, there was plenty of activity, but the nights were long. Instead of worrying, I could be distracted with movies. The laughter and drama kept my mind off my situation, which allowed me to be more calm and even drift into sleep.

Then my parents arrived. That was brutal.

I will never forget the look on my mom's face. She broke down immediately. She was in pure anguish, and all I could say was, "I'm so sorry. I'm so sorry." I just kept apologizing because I knew what I'd done to them, how much I'd scared them, and how I'd changed the rest of their lives.

My dad was stoic as always. He stood there with a blank look on his face. Being a military guy, it's not in his nature to show emotion, especially in a crisis.

As soon as my mom could manage her tears, she began bringing up everything she could think of that needed to be addressed. That's what I love about my mom. She is always ready to anticipate and tackle any challenge. Where was I going to live? Who would take care of me? How would we pay for it all? What kind of care would I need?

These were all important questions, but I wasn't ready to consider them. I just needed to survive the next couple of days. After that, we could begin to address her concerns.

But the fact that she was asking those questions, and worrying about our future, showed me just how much of a burden I would be on my parents. They were already considering how they would care for me.

As soon as my parents were settled in my hospital room, Megan did an emergency run to my house. She knew my mom is a neat freak, and assumed that my house wasn't in the best condition.

Loads of laundry were laying on the floor from the camping trip. My bed was unmade. There was a pile of receipts from the business on the dining room table, and stacks of mail and unpaid bills on the counter. And the kids' rooms were even worse.

My house wasn't always such a mess, but with the break-up with Megan, the state of my house was indicative of my emotional state. My heart was broken and my business was up in the air, and my space was a total mess.

When you leave your house, you never consider that you might not be coming back to it. In my case, I would never be returning as my former self. And now my parents would be seeing my house the way I'd left it.

We don't plan for tragedies. We always think we have more time. And yet we have relatively few days on this earth. My experience taught me to always be prepared while appreciating what we do have. And to ask yourself, if your mother saw your house right now, what would she think?

# CHAPTER 9

# Staring Into the Black

Perhaps one of the things we take for granted the most is the love that comes from our friends and family. In a world of selfishness and greed, there can be no greater blessing than the love and affection of others.

I was so grateful in those first days for all the wonderful people in my life and for the care and love they showed me when they called or visited. So many people came to the hospital that security became annoyed by the extra work my presence was creating for them.

With all the people coming and supporting me, I was aware that other patients in ICU didn't have visitors. I couldn't see them, but I could hear their monitors beeping and their groans and screams of pain. And I couldn't hear any apparent family members and friends consoling them.

But for all the support I had, I still had my inner demons. I had gone from being a self-sufficient man to some who could not take care of his most basic functions without help.

When I started my company, I had every expectation of success. I knew I could overcome any obstacle by meeting with clients and talking through an issue. Suddenly, my head had to be level with my body, I couldn't look at a person talking somewhere else in the room. If my nose itched, someone else had to scratch it. And basic body functions happen whether you feel them or not.

There is an underlying panic that comes when you are that helpless. You understand that if everyone left the room right now, you'd die. I couldn't feel my arms and legs, but my mind was still functioning. I could think all sorts of thoughts, but couldn't move my thumb. I went from a man who did everything for himself, and who helped others, to a totally helpless person. Talk about fear! The panic was always there, just beneath the surface. I was constantly pushing it away. Sometimes that left me more drained than running a race.

And then there was the insomnia. Because my body was healing and morphine was dripping into my veins, I would slumber during the day. Then, when night came, I'd doze for a few minutes, but wake up, wide awake, in the middle of the night. And now, with no one else in the room but Megan sleeping with the chair that would squawk ever few minutes, I would face long hours awake with no one to talk with and no distractions like television. I was reduced to staring at the ceiling, unable to move, but with all sorts of thoughts rampaging through my head.

I called it "staring into the black." My mind would start a downward spiral, thinking of every possible thing that could go wrong. It leaped from one worse-case scenario to the next. It became a spinning black pool. I wanted to sleep, but I couldn't with all the drama cycling through my brain. I faced hour after hour alone in the darkness.

Fortunately, I had Megan at night. Yes, she was asleep, but just hearing her breathing next to me was more comfort than I can describe.

Still, I had no conversations to distract me during the long, dark hours. I couldn't turn on a light to read a book. I couldn't grab my iPod to listen to music. I couldn't flip on the TV to take my mind off the dark. I couldn't move. All I could do was lie there, staring at the ceiling, and let my mind dwell on my help-lessness and worry about my future. Worse, there was a lot of guilt for putting so many people in hardship and pain. Megan didn't plan on a life taking care of a big helpless man. And yet, there she was, sleeping half on my bed and half in the chair. In a few hours she'd have to get ready to go to work.

After several nights of staring in the black, I tried to play a game where I'd look at the flip side. If I was worrying about being able to work and support my family, I'd flip it and ask, "What if I'm completely able to work? What if I'm more suc-cessful than I ever thought I'd be?" If I felt guilty for no longer being able to play basketball with my kids or teaching them to drive, I'd flip it to, "At least I'm going to be there to watch them graduate from high school, get married, and for all their other life events." For every bad thought that came in, I'd ask myself what the opposite side was, and focus on that.

All these years later, I still find myself at night staring into the black. My concerns may be different now, but dread and fear still haunt me at night. The flip side has certainly happened; I'm able to support my family and I'm able to be a part of my chil-dren's lives. And yet, without Megan by my side day in and day out, I still could not survive.

*God bless the caregivers. Caring for another, especially a chronically helpless person, is the most selfless act anyone can do.*

# CHAPTER 10

# **Children**

Tuesday morning, two days after the accident, things changed. The nurse walked in and said, "We're prepping you for surgery."

"Surgery? I thought it was scheduled for Friday."

He shrugged, "It was moved to tomorrow morning."

"Why? What happened?" I asked.

He said, "It's got to be done now."

In that moment, I changed my thoughts about seeing my children. Originally, I didn't want them to see me in the ICU. These parts of the hospital are scary. There is all the extra equipment, and the other patients are also in a bad way. There are screams, and serious nurses and doctors moving quickly between rooms.

Initially, we thought it best to protect Taylor and Christian from all of this. Plus, I figured I would be moved soon to another part of the hospital. It would be quieter there and I'd be in better shape. The visit would be less traumatic.

But now, with all the risks of surgery, I changed my mind. I thought it best to see them before surgery, just in case.

The last time I had seen the kids was waving goodbye to them as they were heading to the movies. And the last time I had spoken to them was when they were in the parking garage and I was preparing to die. A lot had happened in their lives over the last few days. Everyone was distracted and trying to protect them from how bad things really were, but their lives had been turned upside down.

You're not prepared to help your children in a crisis like this. What do you tell them? And when?

Heather wanted to keep the children's lives as routine as possible. She wanted the kids to go to school the day after the accident, but they balked at that. They hadn't had much sleep the night before and their emotions were still raw. So they skipped one day. But then it was back to school, where the teachers, of course, were aware of my situation. The kids got permission to keep their phones turned on, in case something happened to me.

When they arrived at the ICU after school that day, I was surrounded by people. Friends were coming and going, staff were in and out of my room, and I was on medications. I'm chagrined to say, I don't remember the kids visiting me.

I couldn't turn my head to see who was in the room, and they were intimidated by all that was going on around me. And they were scared. Taylor was worried that if Christian freaked out again, she wouldn't be able to protect him because she, too, was overwhelmed by it all.

It's unfortunate that in times like this, children often get overlooked. With so much focus on me and my situation, people had less time for the children. And in our need to protect them, we often left them confused and scared. There aren't manuals on what to do in a situation like this. When is the best time for the kids to see their parent in the hospital? Plus, we couldn't see the future. We didn't know what was going to happen.

It was difficult for them. They were forced into something with little guidance on how to survive it. I would do anything to remove all the pain and confusion my situation has caused them. As the parent. I'm supposed to protect them from such things.

My children have had to deal with so much uncertainty and fear. I'm proud for how well they've done as they've matured into adulthood. I love them so much.

# CHAPTER 11

# Surgery

The evening before surgery, my doctor stopped by to explain why the surgery was moved up. "We have a concern. The disc is pressing on your spine, and that is not good. Also, you have damage to the ligaments in the front of your neck. We need to fuse the spine, and take the disc out, and repair those ligaments."

I asked him, "Am I going to walk again?"

He shrugged, and said nonchalantly, "We'll see."

And with that, he walked out of my room.

I was upset by his response. It was dismissive and not very informative. But in retrospect, it was probably the best thing he could have said.

If he had told me that I wouldn't walk again, which I'm sure was his educated opinion, I would have been discouraged. If he had lied and said, "Yes," I would have resented him later when I found out there was realistically no way I would walk again.

But when he said, "We'll see," it upset me. It made me more determined. I thought, "I'll show him."

Then a nurse came in to shave me. It was the most painful shave ever. I was unable to feel anything from the shoulders down, but they need to shave the one part of my body I can feel—and with a disposable razor. It was torture.

Try having someone shave you while you are laying down with a neck brace on. Of course that didn't work, so they took the neck brace off, which was nerve wracking. Here I was, at risk of being permanently paralyzed, and they were removing my neck brace. What if I flinched when they nicked me?

And her technique wasn't good. The nurse kept shaving against the grain with that dull, cheap razor. To be fair, women don't spend much time shaving faces, but I resented being the one she was practicing on.

And hospitals don't spend money on razors. They get the cheapest things possible. I declared that the guy in purchasing should have to shave with the razors he was buying for the patients.

Seeing this painful scenario play out, my brother jumped in and took over. He, at least, shaved with the grain. And when he was finished, I appreciated the clean feeling I had from having my skin scraped.

But I only had that feeling for a few minutes before they put my brace back on and sedated me. I fell asleep to medications and morphine.

When the morning came, I was in a medicated daze. It was early, but my family was already there. I barely remember that morning. I do remember saying goodbye to my brother and parents before being moved from my bed to the gurney. And I have a vague memory of being wheeled away. And then there was the cold of the operating room with diesembodied voices. There was a three-count as I was moved to another table, and then a mask was placed over my face. I was on another planet, not comprehending what I was going through and what I was facing.

# CHAPTER 12

# After Surgery

When I was next aware of my surroundings, I assumed only a day had passed since my surgery. But it was now Saturday, three days later.

I'd lost three days!

There was a big incision on my neck. My whole neck, upper chest, and jaw were bruised. I was retaining water, so my whole body was swollen. Worse, I couldn't swallow, and I found myself choking on my own saliva. All while suffering the worst thirst ever.

It was the first time since being in the hospital that I thought I wasn't going to make it. I was messed up and miserable. How was it possible that I could continue to live?

I hadn't eaten anything solid in a week, nor had I had anything to drink in days. The slightest amount of saliva caused me to choke to the point of suffocating. I couldn't cough up anything that made it's way into my lungs, and when I started choking, I'd start to throw up. When you're flat on your back, you'll quickly aspirate on even the slightest amount of liquid.

So they had this vacuum tube, like the one your dentist uses, on the wall above my head. Whenever I started choking, Megan or whoever else was in the room would have to grab the suction device and clear everything out of my throat. I had to make a conscious effort to breathe through my nose and spit everything out.

To make matters worse, the tube that was down my throat during surgery had traumatized my epiglottis and kept it open. Which meant that everything that entered my throat went straight into my lungs.

I was constantly choking on mucous draining from my sinuses and then throwing up. If I was alone for even a minute, I might choke to death. Just the thought of it caused me to panic.

Worse, with no water going into my mouth or saliva forming inside my mouth, my tongue was so dry it started to crack. The roof of my mouth felt like an open sore. I began begging for ice chips, something wet, to relieve the pain. The staff told me not to worry, that I was being hydrated by the IV. But that knowledge didn't help the pain in my mouth.

If I lay there, breathing through my nose, quietly concentrating, I was OK. But people asked questions, and I needed to talk. Every time I opened my mouth it caused me to wince in pain.

One nurse went beyond simple assurances about the IV hydrating me. He came up with the idea of wetting a sponge and running it around in my mouth.

It was the first relief I'd had in days. Even if no liquid was making it to the back of my mouth, and certainly none was reaching my throat, just feeling that cool sponge on my tongue and across the roof of my mouth kept me from going insane.

Fortunately, my cousin, Krista, had arrived on Thursday, the day after my surgery. She is a physician who trained at UMC, so she knew the doctors working on me as well as the chief resident. At least I had someone on my side who knew the situation and the people involved. She could advocate for me.

She showed me how swollen my body was. Lying there with my head in a neck brace, unable to move, I couldn't see my body. The steroids had given me edema, which meant I was retaining water. My cousin lifted my arm so I could see my fat hands. My fingers looked like sausages.

I said, "That's not good."

"No it isn't." She began squeezing my fingertips, massaging my hands, and continuing up my arms, trying to get the fluid moving again.

Without her, I'm sure the doctors and staff would have simply shrugged at my swelling body. They were more interested in my injury and how well the surgery had gone.

Doctors and residents continued to come in to discuss me right in front of me as if I wasn't there. They would talk about the physical aspects of my injuries and recovery, while ignoring the mental and emotional side of what I was going through.

I started to insert myself into their conversations, suggesting they ask me about my perspective, what was going on with me physically and emotionally, how they could make me more comfortable.

Now that I was awake from surgery, the hospital staff started getting me ready to be discharged. This was a shock to us. We had been so focused on my accident, surviving it, then going into surgery, we hadn't given much thought to what would happen next. Also, we assumed I would be moved out of ICU into a traditional hospital room once I was stabilized.

It turned out they wanted me out of the hospital, and the staff was focussed on getting me stabilized so they could ship me out. They had two goals before getting rid of me: First, I had to be deemed psychologically fit to leave, and second, I had to be able to swallow on my own.

The psychiatric evaluation was the most insensitive, inane assessment. This lady came in and started asking questions about how I was sleeping, what day it was, and so on. I know she was making sure I wasn't still in a fog from the medications, but how did she think I was sleeping with a burning throat, a cracked tongue, and choking on anything that happened to slip down my throat?

And then she asked, "Are you depressed?"

I answered sarcastically, "Oh, I'm thrilled to be here. I'm enjoying myself immensely. I'm paralyzed, I can't move my body, and I'm going to be relying on others for me the rest of my life. What gives you the idea that I might be depressed?"

She looked at me with an expression of "What?" She had no sense of humor and didn't appreciate my sarcasm.

I don't know if I was depressed or not. What I did know is that I was anxious and upset, uncomfortable, and fearful. And now I was angry at her. I said, "I think we're done here. You can write whatever you've got to write, but I'm going to be okay. You don't have to worry about me."

With that, she left. I felt better when her presence wasn't in the room. How could someone that insensitive be in charge of judging someone's mental health?

But that was the easy part of getting me out of the hospital. The other, getting me to swallow, was not only difficult, it was downright scary.

With me flat on my back, unable to move, and choking every time the tiniest bit of saliva escaped down the back of my throat, how could they test whether or not liquid was making it to my stomach or if it was all ending up in my lungs? I could have told them it was ending up in my lungs, but they needed a way to test it.

So the residents came up with this idea to have me drink a liquid that had barium in it. They could then X-ray me to see if the metal went to my stomach or my lungs.

Of course, the first problem was my head couldn't raise above my chest or I'd become nauseated. My blood pressure would plummet, and I'd pass out.

When you've lain supine as long as I had, and your head hasn't moved to the left or right, the crystals in your inner ear, the ones responsible for balance, settle. Then when you sit up, those crystals begin to swirl, hitting parts of your inner ear that haven't had any stimulation for days. The result is terrible vertigo and nausea. Even after they laid me back down, my head continued to spin.

So, when they said they were going to transfer me to this X-ray machine contraption, I knew it was going to cause me serious discomfort long after their experiment was finished.

They slid me to the side of my bed. Then it took five of them to jostle me to a seated position. Then they swung my legs over the side of the bed. I looked at the distance to the machine and knew there was no way this was medically safe. There would be all sorts of movement on a neck that was operated on just days before.

But they were determined. They swung my body into the machine, but as tall as I am, I didn't fit. They continued to push and prod until they had me crammed in.

Next came this terrible tasting drink. "Okay, now swallow."

I swallowed as instructed, and of course it went straight into my lungs.

There I was, just after surgery, choking uncontrollably, struggling not to throw up while trying to control my panic over not being able to get air into my lungs. All with plummeting blood pressure and no way for me to get back to the safety of my bed without these guys jerking me around.

Still choking, and on the verge of passing out, the residents finally said, "Oh, I don't think this is working. Sorry, we'll have to try this later."

And then came all the movement to get me back into bed, only this time I was choking and almost unconscious.

They concluded they needed to teach me how to swallow before attempting the test again. To do this, they gave me what is called "thick water." This stuff doesn't have any flavor, but it is nasty. It's thick and mucousy. It's the consistency of the biggest loogy you've ever swallowed. As gross as that sounds, thick water is worse.

I thought a better way would be to simply let me suck on some ice chips, but they said no. I had to stay on the thick water until the speech therapist could evaluate me.

Which was Monday morning. The therapist watched me swallow the terrible water and gave her consent. The residents came bumbling backing into the room. I knew what I was in for as soon as I saw them. All the movement and hassle, forcing me into the too-small machine. The nausea. And the terrible tasting drink.

But this time, I swallowed it and didn't choke.

It was progress. And that's when they announced that I would be discharged the next day.

The problem was, I had no where to go.

CHAPTER 13

# Discharged

The hospital's medical staff's main job was to get me out of ICU. If I were not paralyzed, and simply busted up, they would have moved me to a regular hospital bed. But since I was stabilized after surgery, but remained paralyzed, I didn't belong in a traditional hospital room.

Since it is rare for people to be discharged directly from ICU, the hospital had little information and no help for us. They simply had their procedures and seemed to not care what was next for me.

One suggestion was a skilled nursing home. I didn't like the sound of that. Another suggestion was a rehabilitation hospital. But beyond these two options, they provided us with no information about what type of facility we should look for and exactly what kind of care I needed to help me recover.

Where was I supposed to go? What kind of care would I need? What should we look for in a facility? What were the options? What questions should we be asking?

My ad hoc support team went into action, trying to get as much information as possible, as quickly as possible. Cort, my brother, Mom, Dad, Heather, Jeff Marks, Alison Schwartz, and Karen Rogers formed a committee to begin researching what is involved in caring for a quadriplegic. Usually, people in this situation just let things happen to them, but my family and friends are solution-oriented and proactive. They wanted to know what was best for me.

We kept hearing that Craig Hospital is the best spinal cord injury rehab hospital in the country, but it is in Colorado, and we only had a day to figure things out. Yes, I wanted the best, but how would I get to Colorado? What would my family do? It's so far from Vegas that I wouldn't have a support group. I pushed the committee to find something closer to home.

Without any information about what to look for in a rehab facility, they literally Googled "Las Vegas rehab facility" and started there. They printed out the list of names and addresses, and divided it up between them. Then they went out individually to check the different places.

My brother came back and said, "I found this place called Desert Canyon." He handed us brochures while telling us how he'd talked with some of the therapists at the facility. They said they could work with me. But beyond their word and a nice looking brochure, we didn't have much more to go on.

While everyone was in my room, discussing the options, a hospital administrator walked in to announce that I would be discharged in seven hours.

I've never seen my mom yell at someone who was not in the family. But that day, the momma bear came out. "He's just out of surgery. He can't swallow. And you're just going to kick him out onto the street?"

But the administration had their job to do and that was to get me out of their bed as quickly as possible. It was up to me and my family and the support group to figure out the next stage in my recovery.

So we had to make a relatively quick decision, and we chose Desert Canyon. For me, it was nerve wracking. All I'd seen was a brochure. I hadn't talked with anyone. I knew almost nothing about the place. And now I would be spending weeks, if not months, of my life there, entrusting my life to them. But, as I saw it, Desert Canyon was the best choice available to us. So we made the calls.

# CHAPTER 14

# Desert Canyon

At 5:00 PM on Tuesday, May 19, nine days after my accident, the ICU nurses removed my IVs and monitors, transferred me out of my hospital bed onto a gurney, and unceremoniously wheeled me down the hall to the elevator and out the back door where an ambulance waited to take me away.

And that was that. The place where I had all the security of a hospital staff, everything I needed to survive, was now behind me. I was facing a world I knew nothing about and with almost no support from the medial community. I had never been paralyzed before. I didn't know anyone who had gone through what I was going through. Worse, the very people who did have knowledge and experience in this area were more focused on pushing me out their doors than helping me face whatever was next.

The only saving grace about that moment is that I was outside of the hospital. Without movement and most of my sensation gone, I hadn't realized how restrictive the ICU felt. Now, for the first time since the accident, I was outside. Just the feel of fresh air on my skin was relief. And the smells, natural smells that were not laden with cleaning chemicals and the staleness of bodies struggling to survive, were rapturous. This was the first time I had been outside since the accident. The warm summer evening and fresh air was soothing. I could hear "outside" noises like cars, people, birds. Under better circumstances, I would have smiled in relief.

The change of scenery was quick lived as they loaded me into the back of the ambulance. I went from enjoying the sun and the sensations to apprehension. The hospital, for all its problems, had become a safe place for me. And now I was heading into an unknown future.

When I say "ambulance," it wasn't one of the nice trucks you see screaming down the road to save people's lives. This thing was a glorified stationwagon. There was barely enough room for my gurney and me in the back. This vehicle was for transporting people who couldn't sit up, and that was all.

That morning they had cut me off from the morphine I'd been relying on since the accident, so my brain was confused. I couldn't get my bearings and had no sense of direction.

I didn't even know where Desert Canyon was, geographically, so once I was in the ambulance, I tried to figure out where we were driving. I looked out the corners of my eyes for landmarks. I judged the turns we took and calculated the time we travelled between lights. At every stoplight, I'd try to catch sight of a road sign. But nothing looked familiar. If we went around a corner, I tried to visualize where such a corner existed in the Las Vegas Valley. If we went up an incline, I would consider which side of the valley we were on. As hard as I tried, I couldn't get a reference point to judge what direction we were headed.

I was still confused when we slowed and turned into the Desert Canyon complex. I felt the emotions and physical sensations of a young child going to a new school. I was alone in the back, but I knew that Megan and my parents had probably arrived ahead of me.

The back doors opened, and light and fresh air greeted me. Before I was ready, I felt the gurney being pulled out of the ambulance. The wheels dropped. People I didn't recognize were now wheeling me into a structure I had never seen before.

Immediately, I could tell the place was different from the ICU. It seemed nicer and more inviting. It was quieter, people were more relaxed, and I didn't sense the pain that plagued the ICU. I smiled. I was starting the second stage of my journey.

We were greeted by the charge nurse, Rhonda Olsen. She had just arrived on duty and was the first to formally welcome me to the facility.

After I had been transferred from the gurney to my new bed, Rhonda asked me, "Is there anything we can do to make you more comfortable?"

It was a simple, elegant, but extremely powerful question. Up to that point, no one had been concerned about my comfort. In the ICU, they had assumed that because of my spinal injury, I couldn't feel anything; therefore, how could I be uncomfortable? But that wasn't the case.

Because I wasn't eating any solid food, my stomach was producing acid and mucous. This created repeated bouts of diarrhea that were so acidic that my skin was being eaten away. In the ICU, their solution was to put a catheter in my rectum. It was extremely uncomfortable.

When Rhonda asked about my comfort, the only thing I could think about was the catheter. And since modesty goes out the window when you're paralyzed, I said, "You can get whatever is in my butt pulled out because it doesn't feel good."

Rhonda chuckled and said, "If you can feel that, it's a good sign."

I said, "It's fantastic that it is a good sign, but it still doesn't feel good. So if you can work on getting that out, that'd be great."

She patted my arm, "I will talk to the doctor."

As a new admit, they had to set a baseline for me. So three nurses set to work to take my vitals, having me blow into a tube to test the strength of my lungs, and checking me for bed sores. In the process, they'd flip me to my right and then to my left, looking at my heels, elbows, even between my butt cheeks. I laughed, thinking I'd have to make the best of the examination.

Since there wasn't anything for me to do while they looked over, I asked them if they had any music. I hadn't heard any music since the day of the accident, and I love music. They turned on a little bedside mono-speaker. They dialed through the channels. I had a choice between Muzac, easy listening, adult contemporary, and Motown. I chose Motown. When "Heard it through the Grapevine" came on, I started singing and the nurses joined in. They knew at that moment that I wasn't going to be the usual spinal injury patient.

Next, they set to work to clean me up. I hadn't had a bath in nine days. My hair was dirty. You don't think of it, but your hair actually hurts when it is that dirty. Much to my dismay, I found out they would not be able to wash my hair because I was not allowed to have my neck brace taken off and they didn't want to get the incision in my neck wet. All they could do was pat my face with a damp washcloth and use dry shampoo on my hair. The dry shampoo wasn't satisfying, but at least I didn't feel so dirty.

By then, Rhonda was back with good news. They could remove the colon catheter. She reiterated that if I could feel the catheter, it was a good sign.

I asked why, and she said "It's an indication that your pelvic shelf is going to come back."

"What's a pelvic shelf? Do you place awards on it?"

She smiled and explained that it is what controls the ability to sense if your bladder is full or if you are going to have a bowel movement, and the fact that I could feel my colon meant that my pelvic shelf might come back. And if that could come back, maybe other things could come back as well.

With that assurance, I felt thankful for the discomfort the colon catheter was causing me. It meant I was on my way to recovery. Of course, I felt even better when they removed it.

# CHAPTER 15

# Taking Charge

After all the activity of that first day at Desert Canyon, Megan and I were looking forward to the first peaceful night we'd had in a long time. Instead of sleeping in the chair by my bed, Megan now had an actual cot. And we were no longer surrounded by the beeps and screams that plague the nights in ICU. I was clean and comfortable.

But the peaceful night I had hoped for lasted until 3:00 AM. I woke up and did what I always did, all I could do, and that was stare into the black.

I realized nights were still going to be an insidious form of torture. My body clock was off. During the days, I would struggle with uncontrollable deep naps, but at night, I'd be wide awake for hours on end with nothing to do, no one to talk to, just alone with my thoughts, worries, and fears.

Of course, I eventually fell asleep just before the rest of the hospital woke up. I struggled to awaken as the nurses began their rounds, distributing medications. Then the breakfast tray arrived, and all I wanted to do was sleep.

That first morning, the medical director, Dr. Merle Burman, came in to introduce himself and to look me over. He was soft-spoken, short, and balding.

Over the next few weeks, we struck up an odd relationship. His personality is the exact opposite of mine. He is very analytical and serious compared to my humor and gregariousness. I called him "the Burmanator," and he wouldn't crack a smile.

Dr. Burman caught on early that he wasn't going to get anything by us. We had questions, lots of questions. We wanted to know what was going on and what we could expect. We weren't going to let him sneak in at 6:30 AM and take a quick look at my chart.

We had learned from our experience at ICU that we had to be vigilant with the doctors and nurses. We learned to question everything so that we would know what was happening and why it was being done.

Too often, patients automatically accept what the medical staff say to them. The reality is that you should pay more attention to your situation than the medical staff does. Yes, people like Dr. Burman and most of the staff at the hospital care about their patients and job, but they have many other patients to consider. They may not take the time to think through specific options for you.

Unfortunately, you will get people who aren't dedicated to their jobs or their patients. For instance, there was one nurse who wasn't diligent with my medications, which was a rather important part of her job.

I have a pharmaceutical background, so I would make the nurses show me the cup of meds before taking them. If I saw one I hadn't seen before, I'd ask about it.

A few days after checking into Desert Canyon, I saw a pill I didn't recognize. I said, "That's a different pill. What is it?"

The nurse said, "It's a stool softener."

I hadn't had solid food in over a week. Anything coming out of me was bile and stomach fluid. I said, "You don't understand, I'm supposed to be taking medication that will keep me from having diarrhea."

She looked down and said, "Oh, those are room 309's pills." I was in room 307.

On another day, the same nurse handed me my medication, and once again there were a couple pills I didn't recognize. "What's that?" I asked

She said, "That's your hypertension medication," meaning the pills were meant to lower my blood pressure. But Dr. Burman was trying to *raise* my blood pressure. I had been lying down for so long that my blood pressure was already dangerously low.

"What? Are you guys are trying to kill me!" I exclaimed.

When Dr. Burman heard about the situation, he fired the nurse on the spot. That was two times she'd messed up my medications in three days. If I hadn't looked or questioned her, I would have died.

You have to manage your own care when you're in the hospital. You have to hold your healthcare providers accountable. Don't assume they have the same dedication to their job that you do to your own life and health.

In my case, this was even more important because I was dependent on the people around me for everything. A slight slip-up, even a bout of forgetfulness, and I could die.

We also had to figure the best ways to care for me. Unlike the ICU, the nurses were now a long ways away from me, and I couldn't push the call button to summon them.

I was still having problems swallowing, and the threat of choking to death was still very real.

We had the same set up with the oral vacuum above my bed, but if there were no nurses within earshot, they wouldn't hear me choking.

For some reason, no one thought about how a paralyzed person would call a nurse. Yes, there are devices you can blow into, but if you can't move your hands, how do you get the device to your mouth?

Working with the medical staff, we rigged a button so that it was wedged under my neck brace. If I shrugged my left shoulder just right, it would activate the button. While it only worked half the time, I can't tell you how relieved I was that I had at least a shot to call a nurse if no one was in the room.

Taking responsibility for your own healthcare doesn't just protect you from the oversights and slip-ups of others, but it also gives you a sense of empowerment. Instead of lying helplessly, blindly going through the routines caregivers set up for you, you have a sense of involvement in your progress. You can empower yourself by simply asking "why."

# CHAPTER 16

# Physical Therapy

As Dr. Burman finished our first consultation, he mentioned that the next thing on my schedule was physical therapy.

"Physical therapy," I thought. "What are they going to do? Teach me how to blink my eyes?" I was seriously confounded over how you rehab a body that can't move. I looked up at the ceiling and let out a heavy sign, and thought, "God, how am I going to do this?"

Then I heard a person walk into my room. They leaned over my bed and came into my line of sight. I was surprised to see a woman with big brown eyes. She couldn't have been more than 5'3" and 105 pounds dripping wet.

She said in a conversational whisper, "Hi, I'm Deborah Howell. I'm going to be your physical therapist."

She paused, but I didn't have a reply, still wondering what we were going to do for therapy. I thought, "I'm a big guy, I can't move. How's this tiny thing going to rehab me?"

As if reading my mind, Deborah straightened up and spoke in a commanding tone, "Ninety percent of what you get back will be from effort and attitude. Ten percent will be nature. Is that clear?"

Talk about hearing the right message at the right time. In those few words, she gave me the most inspiring sermon. I understood that my recovery would be directly proportional to my effort and attitude, two things I still had one hundred percent control over. I realized that God had just answered my prayer. I now knew how I was going to do this. It would take a strong effort and a great attitude.

I looked in her expressive eyes and said, "We're not going to have a problem. Push me as hard as you can, as long as it is medically safe. If we can stretch sessions, stretch them. If we can add an extra session, add them. I'll do whatever it takes to walk out of this place."

I hadn't meant to say anything about walking out of the hospital; in fact, I hadn't even had that thought until I spoke it aloud. It was my first audacious goal, and it became my battle cry: "Walk out of this place."

You've heard the saying, "If you shoot for the stars, you can settle for the moon." Without audacious goals, you have nothing to shoot for. When we are complacent, satisfied with where we are, we won't have the inspiration nor the perseverance needed to achieve an audacious goal.

For me to walk, I would need to work hard getting my muscles and the rest of my body ready. Simply lying on my back and complaining about my lot in life would not yield the miracle of walking out of the hospital. And it all starts with attitude. Once we adopt an attitude of expectation, and are willing to put forth a corresponding effort, amazing things will happen.

So my therapy started that day. There was no resting, no getting settled. We were on a path to success, and there wasn't any time to waste.

Of course, we began with an assessment of where I was physically. There was about an hour of, "Do you feel this? Can you move that? Try this." Deborah moved different joints to see what strength and mobility I had left. At the end of our session, she didn't give me any bad news, just encouragement that we were in a good place to begin therapy.

Years later, Deborah told me, "When we saw your chart and reviewed it before coming in to meet you, we decided we'd be satisfied if we could get you to move your hands so you could operate an electric wheelchair, maybe feed yourself. That was our goal before meeting you."

Hearing that, I'm glad that the audacious goal of walking out of the facility blurted out of my mouth. It let Deborah know that I could take whatever she threw my way. I wanted to succeed, and I needed her help.

Little did I know, she could dish it out. After all, Deborah was *Retired Navy Captain* Deborah Howell.

Our first goal in therapy was to be able to sit upright. You can't begin to rehab unless you can sit upright for an extended period of time. At that point, if my upper-body was even slightly elevated, I'd get nauseated and struggle to stay conscious.

When you have a head or spine injury, the response of your parasympathetic, or "involuntary," nervous system is to lay you down. Since the time we were cavemen, when we took a blow to the head, our bodies would not let us stand until we had begun to heal. So your body drops your blood pressure to make you pass out. Even if I had wanted to sit up, and even if I had control of my muscles to hold my body upright, my parasythetic nervous system, sensing my spine injury, wanted me flat on my back.

Deborah began by raising the head of my bed with the electronic controls. I could hear the whirring of the motor as my head was raised above the level of my chest. Deborah would watch me and monitor my blood pressure. When it was clear that I could tolerate an angle, she'd raise me a little more.

Suddenly my nervous system would say, "Time to lay you down," and my blood pressure would plummet. I would begin to pass out. I felt as though I was about to vomit. Deborah would then quickly lower my bed and let me get my wits about me. Then she'd raise the bed again.

It may sound easy having her raising me up and lowering me back down, but it was a lot of work for me. We were retraining my sympathetic, or "voluntary," nervous system to take over my parasympathetic nervous system.

The simple struggle to stay conscious and not throw-up while being raised a few degrees and then lowered back down was more exhausting than any physical exertion I'd experienced before the accident. It was the strangest thing to be so worn out when I hadn't moved a muscle.

It was then that I grasped how long of a journey I was in for. It was easy to say, "I'm going to walk out of here." But experiencing how difficult it was to have them raise me up a few degrees made the goal seem impossible. The panic crept up inside. I couldn't breathe. I was scared because I didn't think I could do this.

# CHAPTER 17

# Be the Hope

In the middle of my exhaustion and depression over how far I had to go, my parents and a couple nurses came into my room with a cupcake that had a birthday candle in it.

My mom realized that we had missed my birthday the previous Sunday. That had been the day that we discovered I would be discharged from ICU, and everyone was scrambling to figure out where I would go.

Now that I was safely at Desert Canyon, my mom thought it would be good to celebrate a few days late.

But when I saw that small cupcake and heard them singing, I thought, "Are you kidding me? Happy Birthday? What's happy about it?" I still could not swallow without choking, so I couldn't eat the cupcake. I couldn't even raise my head high enough to blow out the candle.

As I had these thoughts, I suddenly realized they were eagerly watching for my reaction. I refocused. I knew that how

I reacted would affect those who love me and care for me. If I was down because this was the worse birthday ever, they would also be down. They were looking for emotional direction from me. If I let on how pathetic the whole situation seemed to me, they would also feel bad, and they'd feel ashamed for putting together this thoughtful birthday celebration.

I quickly thought, "What would the opposite reaction look like?" Instead of projecting sadness, I could project hope. It's then that I came up with what would become my new mantra, "Be the hope."

I enthusiastically finished the happy birthday song with them by singing , "Happy birthday to me... And many more."

As if they read my mind, they held the cupcake with the candle near my lips, below my chin. I gave it a puff downward, but it didn't blow out. I gave it another puff. Quickly, one of the nurses blew the candle out, and they all clapped triumphantly for me.

From that point on, when people came into my room, I would joke about my stunt bike career being short-lived. Or, I'd say things like, "At least now I won't have to fold another load of laundry or even tie my shoes."

My jokes surprised people, but also set them at ease, letting them know that we could talk lightly and frankly about my injury.

It was important for me that people feel comfortable when they visited me, so they would keep coming back. If they felt awkward and left depressed, they'd start to find reasons not to come by. So, I was determined to be the hope.

I discovered there are two sides of the equation. It wasn't just about making sure that people took care of me, I had to make sure that I was caring for them as well.

A patient in my situation must realize they have to be kind to and supportive of their caregivers. No one wants to take care of a jerk or someone wallowing in self-pity. The dependent one must inspire people. When you're pleasant, nurses will check in on you more often, physical therapists will work with you harder, doctors will take the time to explain to you what is going on.

Yes, my situation was difficult and at times hopeless, but I was also dependent on a lot of people: nurses, therapists, friends, and family. If I focused on being the hope, it made taking care of me that much easier. I would be less of a burden both physically and emotionally, and maybe even uplift and inspire them.

Being helpless doesn't mean we need to be hopeless.

# CHAPTER 18

# The Message

It had been a long and difficult day. My seemingly inconsequential first day of therapy had left me physically and emotionally exhausted. I wanted to go to sleep early in the evening, which was rare for me. I simply didn't want to think about my situation any more. So with Meg in the cot beside me, I quickly fell asleep.

And I slept hard for five hours, waking up a little after 2:00 AM. I could hear Megan breathing rhythmically next to me. While I stared straight up, the room closed in on me. I slipped quickly into "staring into the black." The swirling pool of "what ifs," bitter thoughts, and angry feelings welled up. Why did this happen to me? Why?

Suddenly I heard a voice. It was weird. It was as if the voice was coming from inside of me. But I could hear it as clear as if someone were talking to me from the foot of my bed.

It said, "All you have wanted to do your whole life was dance, when all I have wanted you to do was sing. You can no longer dance, but you can sing. Witness to my power, and you will be healed."

It scared me. It wasn't my internal voice, and there was no one in the room except for Megan. My heart raced. And then I stopped and thought about the words.

That voice was concise. More telling, it was the perfect metaphor for me. My life had been about the party, about the pursuit of my own selfish desires. My life was about me "dancing."

And now I no longer had my ability to dance. But what did I still have? My voice. I could "sing." I had sung in a garage band back in college; I was awful. So, I was pretty sure the voice didn't want me to pursue a career in singing. What it meant by "singing," referenced my ability to speak, persuade, and inspire.

The phrase, "witness to my power," were not words I would have consciously constructed. It dawned on me that I was hearing the voice of God. It was a commandment.

I had often used my gift to "sing" for selfish and destructive pursuits. I was always one to talk people into having one more drink, staying out one more hour, and not caring about tomorrow. Everyone loved me for that. But when had I ever used my ability to "sing" to share the faith I'd been raised in? I had wasted a lot of opportunities.

The majority of my life, I'd chosen to resist God for control. He was always there, right next to me, quietly asking me to submit to His guidance and sing His song. Instead, I would ignore Him, and continue dancing.

"Meg," I called out. "Meg."

She struggled awake, "What's wrong?"

I said, "God's here. In this room."

She said, "What?"

"God is here, in this room with us."

As I told her about the message, I became acutely aware that my pride and arrogance had gotten in God's way. I knew I was being hard on myself, but if God was speaking to me that directly, I needed to listen. I knew that I'd disappointed Him, but I also knew He still loved me and wanted the best for me.

With tears streaming from my eyes, pooling behind my ears, I bitterly admitted how ashamed I was. "Every time I've been given an opportunity to walk the right path, I've danced to my own tune. I've rebelled against what God wanted me to do. I've squandered my gift to "sing."

Meg reached across my body to hug me. She wiped the tears from my face and kissed me gently on my cheek. She told me that she loved me.

Pondering the message, Meg and I eventually fell asleep.

As the hospital awoke several hours later, I could still hear God's words. The awesomeness of His message hadn't diminished with the light of morning. But now there was a change. Instead of feeling ashamed for how I had been in the past, oddly, I found myself excited for my future.

# CHAPTER 19

# The Healing

In the morning, Megan went to work and I faced another round of physical therapy. The elation I'd felt from God's message diminished as physical exhaustion took over.

As soon as Deborah announced that the session was over, I was asleep in a manner that I'd later term a "power coma." My exhaustion would be so complete, and my body's struggle to heal so immense, that I would fall into a sleep so deep that when I'd wake, I'd swear a lifetime had passed. These "comas" were way more than any nap I'd experienced before.

When I awoke that afternoon, struggling to come back to consciousness, I saw Heather, my ex-wife, next to me. It took me a couple minutes to realize who was with her, an ex-business associate, Paul Henry.

I was shocked to see him. Of all the people who could or would visit me, I never anticipated that Paul would be standing next to my bed at that moment.

Two years earlier, a business deal had gone wrong. I felt that Paul had taken advantage of me. The last thing I'd said to him was, "You are no friend of mine!"

And now here he was in my room. While Paul and I did go way back, there were times we would have slugged each other if we were in the same room. The hatchet may have been buried, but it was still within reach.

And now that there was nothing physically I could do to protect myself, Paul was in my room, looking down on my helpless body.

Paul touched my shoulder and said, "Scott, I want to pray on you."

I was so stunned by the situation, I didn't respond. Why would Paul Henry want to pray on me? Why would he want to pray with me at all?

Thinking back to the message from the night before, I relented. I noticed he said, "pray on," not "with." But I thought, "I'm up for anything."

In the days since the accident, I'd had several people come in and pray with me. Theirs were traditional prayers, like the Lord's Prayer, or something similar to, "Father, please heal your son, Scott, and make him feel better..." I'd also been put on various prayer chains.

And while I wasn't praying much at that point in my life, I wasn't resistant to expressions of faith that other people showed on my behalf. In fact, I was comforted and honored by all those prayers.

But Paul? It was awkward. But I thought, "If someone wants to pray for me, let them."

Out of the corner of my eye, I saw my father, Randy, was also in the room. He didn't know the history between Paul and me. And while my father is a church man, he does not express his faith. You won't hear him witness or even talk about his religion.

I knew that my dad would be comfortable with a traditional prayer for me, but anything more than that would make him uneasy. Which is why I worried a bit when Paul gathered everyone around my bed and asked them to hold hands.

Paul started with the usual prayer, but then he veered into speaking a strange language. While I was trying to figure out what was going on, Paul began moving his hands over my body, not touching me, just hovering his hands an inch or two above me.

He'd break from his strange gibberish and say, "Heather, pray for Scott for healing." And then, "Randy, say a prayer."

All of this was counter to my father's religious experience. It's difficult for him to pray aloud, much less deal with someone speaking a strange language and floating his hands around. Heather stepped up when my dad faltered and continued praying aloud.

When there was a pause in Heather's prayers, Paul would tell me to keep my eyes shut and let God in and keep Him in my heart.

This went on for 20 minutes. The tension in the room was palpable. Just as I was getting ready to tell Paul to stop, I started to get a warm sensation. It started moving from my chest into my limbs. With my eyes still closed, I saw a purple light, kind of like an old screen-saver. I could hear Paul's voice reaching a crescendo in the strange language, and I could sense his hands hovering over my chest.

Then his hands touched me. At that moment, electricity shot through me. He said, "Father show us a sign that you are going to heal your son, Scott. Show us a sign we cannot refute. Do it now."

At that instant, I felt like I was convulsing. I opened my eyes and looked down at my feet. My legs got stiff. Then they lifted about five inches off the bed and stayed there a couple of seconds. It wasn't like I was doing a leg lift; instead, it felt like someone was lifting my feet off the bed for me.

When my legs dropped back down to the bed, I looked sideways at my dad. He physically stumbled backwards, lifting his hands up like he was going to be burned by what he saw. This was definitely not something he'd seen before, and certainly outside the military/academic world.

Paul took a deep breath. He was sweating. He looked at me and said, "Do you have any doubt you are going to be healed?"

I didn't know what to say. Even with all that had just happened, there was this part of me that was trying to figure it out. This was a guy I hadn't had a lot of connection to, a person I didn't like, and he had done this for me. I stammered, and finally mumbled, "No doubt."

From that point on, I stopped soft-shoeing my spirituality. When people said, "Let's pray," I prayed. When people said, "I hope you get better." I said, "With God's power, I will." With each little progress I had, I'd say, "Praise be to God."

With God visiting me the night before, and my encounter with Paul the next day, I clearly heard God's message, "Tell people about me. Use your gift. Sing." I started making a conscious effort to tell people I was going to be healed and God would help.

# CHAPTER 20

# Mom's Touch

Word of Paul's visit traveled quickly. Friends, family, and even the hospital's staff were talking about it.

My dad, as stoic as he is, was telling anyone who would listen to the story and how he had wanted to say, "hallelujah" when he saw my legs move.

When I heard him say that, I chided him, "Dad, that would have been a perfect time to say *hallelujah*."

Later that afternoon, I was working in occupational therapy, trying to move my hand. Suddenly, my left thumb did something it hadn't done in weeks—it began to move. Ever so slightly, I could rotate my thumb toward the palm of my hand.

It was the first real evidence that I could recover movement. I was giddy with my accomplishment. I kept showing people how I could move my thumb that little bit.

When my mom heard about Paul's visit, she rushed to the hospital. I showed her my new stunt. Just like when I was seven, jumping off the diving board, I said, "Mom, watch." And I slowly rotated my thumb back and forth for her.

She grabbed my left hand and said, "Squeeze my hand."

For the first time, I realized that I was feeling her hand grasping mine. There isn't anything more powerful than feeling your mother's touch, especially after weeks of her touching me and me not feeling anything.

I wanted, with all my spirit, to show her how much the feel of her holding my hand meant to me. I looked down, focused, and suddenly my fingers began to move. She stared down at my tightening fingers and began to cry.

I told her, "This is just the beginning."

I knew that she was beginning to believe that miracles were about to happen. She now had the hope that her son would not be as helpless as he now was, that maybe she would witness him standing and walking some day.

For me, the feeling of her touch and the realization that the sensation in my fingers was returning was overwhelming. I began to cry, thankful for the miracle. These small movements would be the beginning of many accomplishments and miracles yet to come. It was time to prepare for the possible.

# CHAPTER 21

# The Little Things

Despite the most recent miracles, the reality of life quickly returned. I was still stuck in bed, and would be for weeks and months to come.

Anyone who's been in a hospital bed knows you've got the up/down button for your legs and head. You also have a speaker on a cord for your television, and you've got some music channels that come out of this static mono-speaker.

At least we had basic cable. After all, the NBA playoffs were on, and I needed a diversion. Even before the accident, I would have spent every game glued to the television, especially with the Lakers in the playoffs; now, however, I couldn't pull myself away from the television if I wanted to.

The problem was I still couldn't have my bed raised up for any length of time, and the television was set about head high on the opposite wall.

One of the nurses, Scott Ryan, understood how important the NBA playoffs were for me. He also understood, it would be dangerous to raise my bed to watch the game. Plus, I would miss key plays if I passed out. So he set to work to solve the problem.

He unplugged everything, got out a step ladder, moved the cords around, and finally placed the television on top of the armoire. Up there, the television was almost touching the ceiling. And while it still wasn't the best angle, I could look out the bottom of my eyes and see the game on the distant, small television.

It wasn't like watching at home, or at the local sports bar, but at least I didn't miss a single game that season.

It was a small gesture that meant the world to me. And the games were a welcome break from the gruelling physical therapy sessions.

Once Deborah caught on to how important the playoffs were to me, she saw another opportunity to torture me. She said that if I wanted to watch the game, I would have to turn on the TV by myself. And I had to change the channels to the station I wanted. At that point, I could only squeeze with my left hand, so she at least had the mercy to put the remote in that hand.

But I didn't have the ability to press with my thumb, which you need with a remote. I also wasn't able to lift my left arm to point the remote at the television.

The game started at 6:00 PM, and it was now 6:07, and I was struggling. Eventually, Deborah positioned the remote so it was pointing up at the television so that I would have a chance at turning the TV on and finding the right channel.

That was learning dexterity the hard way. The more minutes I missed of the game, the more motivated I got. It was a relief when the television finally turned on, but of course it was on the wrong channel.

A good 15 minutes was lost by the time I managed to get my thumb on the channel up button, pressing as hard as I possibly could to advance to the right channel.

When I heard the announcers talking about the game, I was happy that I hadn't missed much. I threw Deborah an angry look for making me struggle.

She just smiled and patted me on the shoulder, "See you tomorrow."

"I can't wait," I said sarcastically. Privately, though, I celebrated my achievement as I began to enjoy the game.

The problem for me was that any distractions that might be present during the day, like the playoffs, weren't available at night.

Most of the patients were older, having suffered from strokes, hip and knee surgeries, and the like. So after about 10:00 PM, when everyone had taken their meds, things got really quiet in the hospital.

I'm a night owl, and since there wasn't much for the nurses to do at night, they'd come by and visit with Megan and me. We'd usually be up past midnight, visiting with them.

I remember one night in particular. The nurses had left and Megan and I were watching television. She was dead tired from working all day, so she fell asleep before the first show had finished.

A Chuck Norris movie marathon was on AMC. The little mono-speaker was four inches from my right ear, and it was two clicks too high in volume to allow me to drift off to sleep. And Megan was now fast asleep.

Movie after movie played, and no one came in to check on me. Because Megan was with me, I didn't have my call button hooked up. All I could do was stare with near-unconsciousness at the challenges Chuck Norris faced. Kick after kick, lame line after lame line, punches that landed with loud thuds, and breaking glass stretched in a long succession throughout the night.

When the *The Octagon* came on, I smiled with a memory of how I can gone to see the movie in the theater as a child. I anticipated all the wonder I felt back then. But as the movie unwound, I thought, "Man, I wasted my five bucks back then."

When finally the Chuck Norris catalogue was exhausted, AMC switched to Vincent Price's original version of *The Fly*, which was better than the Chuck Norris films, but only just.

I remember seeing the sky lighten out of the corner of my eye, and sighing in relief. I'd survived the night of Chuck Norris and Vincent Price. But I was exhausted.

With the shift change, a nurse finally came to check on me. "Could you please turn off the TV," I croaked.

It was one of the longest nights of my life. The only thing that saved me was knowing that Megan had gotten a full night of restful sleep.

As for me, I hope I never see a Chuck Norris movie again.

# CHAPTER 22

# Sitting Upright

A few days later, I was able to tolerate Deborah raising up my bed so that my head was well above my chest. This meant I was ready for the next stage in my physical therapy, which was a whole new kind of torture.

I couldn't move my arms yet, and my muscle tone was greatly diminished. When I was sitting upright, my arms would hang heavy from my shoulders. You could literally see the ball of my shoulder joints pulling out of their sockets. And since I had feeling from my chest up, the pain of slow dislocation was almost more than I could handle. If you've had someone crank your arm behind your back, you know a little bit about the pain I was experiencing. Worse, there was nothing I could do to relieve it.

Two nurses had to help Deborah sit me up. First, they'd put compression hose on my legs to force blood out of my legs and back to my core, thus keeping my blood pressure up. The hose were super tight, so it took forever for the nurses to stretch them over my long, unresponsive legs.

Next, they'd put a straight-jacket type contraption on my upper body to brace my arms. These braces had handles that kept my arms half-bent, removing some of the strain on my shoulders. But the nurses still had to position my arms to keep my shoulders in their sockets.

When they were finally ready to get me upright, they rolled me on my side, and with two nurses behind me, lifting, Deborah moved my legs over the bed. Everyone held me in position waiting for my blood pressure to drop. They'd time me with a stop watch: 15 seconds, 30 seconds, 45 seconds. Then we would hit the point where I started to lose consciousness, and they'd carefully lower me back down.

I'd lay on my back, panting, fighting to gain control. When I could calm down enough, we'd start the whole process again. Then I'd start to pass out, and it was back down. Before I was totally recovered, they'd roll me on my side and begin lifting me. Again and again, we did this until the therapy session was finished.

It was exhausting.

After a couple days attempting this feat, Deborah concluded, "We've got to get you on a tilt table."

"What's a tilt table?"

"It's exactly what it sounds like."

Well, not exactly. It's more like a big hand truck/bed combination. It looks like a prop for a Frankenstein movie. It's what they would use to take the monster to get electrocuted. It has a foot plate on the bottom, big straps for the shins, thighs, and chest. All that was missing was an angry crowd with pitch forks.

They rolled it next to my bed and four people gathered around to transfer me. On three, they moved me onto the board. Next, all the straps where stretched and locked down.

The advantage was that my whole body could tilt, instead of sitting me on the side of my bed. It was easier and faster to elevate me and lay me back down when I was about to pass out.

The goal was to simulate being in the standing position. But we didn't want to get to 90 degrees, because I'd slip out of the harness. Instead, the goal was 75 degrees. At that angle, organs shift. You don't notice it or think about it when you are an able-bodied person, but when you stand, your organs shift involuntarily. But when you've been on your back for a long time, any shift in your organs causes all sorts of nerve responses that once again cause you to pass out to keep the movement from continuing.

So they'd crank me to 20 degrees and wait for me to get control. Then they'd move me to 30 degrees. The problem was, I couldn't close my eyes even though that is our natural reaction when we get vertigo. The only way I could progress was to keep my eyes open and breathe deeply. I'd find a focal point and stare at it, trying to get control of my body.

That's when I came up with the idea of playing music while I was going through this torture. I said, "We've got to have a playlist to help take my mind off the nausea. I can rock out while fighting it."

So we put together my "Tilt-table Playlist." It started with the Killers *All These Things I've Done*. The song appropriately starts with "I want to stand up. I want to let go." We also had U2's *Beautiful Day*, Bruce Springstein's *Born in the USA*. I needed fighting songs, protest songs, life-sucks-and-we're-pushing-through songs. When they rolled in the tilt-table, I knew the next hour was going to be rough. And I needed to fight back.

The playlist also became a timing mechanism. My goal was to make it all the way through a song at 20 degrees. Then make it half way through the next song at 30 degrees, and so on.

The worst part of the struggle was that when your organs shift, you often have a colic reflex, that's a fancy way of saying I would poop my pants. And since I was strapped in, we couldn't stop to clean me up. I had to keep going. I could only make jokes about how I was no longer full of crap. Or I'd say, "Houston, we have a rear-hatch malfunction."

By making jokes, it made the staff feel more comfortable about pushing me. The more I could take, the more they would push. There was a lot of laughing on that tilt-table. I don't remember that being part of Frankenstein's monster's struggle.

Whenever we face struggles, it's best to divert our attention. Without diversions, we focus on the ordeal, what we're feeling and facing. But with music and humor, my attention was focussed on success. I could do a better job fighting my body's natural responses.

# CHAPTER 23

# True Love

Megan's life was getting a little easier now that she could sleep through most of the night. Granted, she still didn't have a proper bed. Then I'd keep her up late and the nurses began their rounds early in the morning. But at least she wasn't half sitting/half lying in a chair that squawked every few minutes.

One evening, they had me propped on my side. I looked over at her. I could see her struggling with exhaustion. She'd been through so much with me these last couple of weeks, especially when you factor in the pain I'd caused her before the accident. I became overwhelmed in that moment, realizing how unworthy I was for her dedication and love.

"Megan, this is going to take so long, and I don't know what's going to happen. I don't want to be a burden."

She started to shake her head, but I continued, "You don't have to do this. You are young. You could have a full and wonderful life."

I paused, "You don't have to do this. I don't want you to feel obligated to be here for the rest of your life."

She didn't bat an eye, "I love you, who you are. I'm not going anywhere."

I fell in love with her all over again.

We didn't talk about our relationship from that point on. We each understood that we were back together. If she was going to dedicate her life to me, then I would try my hardest to be the best person I could be for her.

People always say what an angel Megan is, and they are right, but my response is, "What am I? Chopped liver?"

Megan didn't choose to be with me just to be miserable. We are a partnership. We love each other. Just as she cares for me, I strive to be deserving of that care.

Megan has a nurturing gene. She likes to take care of people. That is why God brought her into my life during the chaotic time after my divorce and when I took custody of my children. Maybe God also knew what was in store for me, and He made sure this miracle was positioned well in advance, so that when I needed her, Megan was there.

# CHAPTER 24

# Second Healing

Since I'd last seen Paul, my thumb had started to move, I'd squeezed my mother's hand, I'd worked hard on the tilt table, and was beginning to tolerate it better. My big toe had recently started to move, and I could bend my right elbow. All good signs. But I'd be lying if I'd said the process wasn't wearing on me. And I was still struggling to sit up on the side of the bed for longer than a minute.

My ex-wife, Heather, brought Paul back to visit me. Again, he said he wanted to pray on me. This time there was no hesitation from me. I was excited to see what was going to happen.

Between his last visit and this one, I had discovered that Paul had adopted the Pentecostal faith and had acquired the ability to speak in tongues. Paul was not shy about his faith, to the point that it had begun to alienate him from his business associates. He didn't seem to mind. He loved being able to channel God's power.

Paul could sense my enthusiasm, but before he started to pray, he rested a hand on my shoulder and asked, "What is it you fear?"

An elegant, short, powerful question. I stammered, not knowing where to start. There is a lot to fear in modern life: How to pay bills, threat of job loss, rejection by loved ones. And here I was dependent on others for even the basics of life. Needless to say, there was a lot for me to fear.

Then he asked, "Do you believe you are going to be healed?"

I said, "Yes, but I fear that I don't have what it takes." I then told him that while believed I would be healed, I wasn't sure if it would be quick enough or if I had the mental fortitude to sustain the effort necessary to rehab my entire body.

He said, "So let's pray to speed it up."

Then he began the same ritual as before. Paul asked the people in the room to join hands and begin praying for me. Again, it made them uncomfortable watching Paul speaking in tongues and laying hands on me.

Suddenly, the same thing began happening as before. A warmth radiated from my chest through my limbs. The spiraling purple light returned behind my eyes. And Paul's crescendo of words flooded my being.

Paul paused in his strange language and said, "Father, show us an irrefutable sign." But nothing happened.

Paul looked at me and said, "Do you believe?"

I said, "Yes," but I could tell he sensed doubt in me.

He said, "Scott, you've got to believe."

I responded, "I do."

He shot me a sideways glance. "I don't think you do."

Paul went on to tell me, "The first time I was here, I expected you to get up and walk. That's the kind of faith you have to have, Scott."

Paul waited, and then said, "Let me know what happens."

# CHAPTER 25

# The Recovery Speeds up

The next morning, Deborah came in for therapy. We went through the usual ritual of putting on the hose, then the straight-jacket, and finally the nurses pushed me into a seated position as Deborah swung my legs over the edge of the bed. The blood pressure cuff was monitoring me, and Deborah started the stop watch.

And, as before, we waited for the nausea and faintness. Deborah watched me, waiting.

One minute passed, and we were still looking at each other. The nurses behind me relaxed a bit.

Then two minutes passed, and I was not throwing up or feeling like I was going to pass out.

Then three minutes passed. The tension began to rise between us.

I was startled when the opening song in my mix finished and I was still sitting upright.

Suddenly, I had the realization that I could feel my stomach muscles. But I didn't say anything in case the feeling went away.

Deborah kept looking at my vitals and into my eyes, waiting for me to succumb.

I became aware that a third song had started. Does this mean we are coming on ten minutes?

Then a fourth song started to play.

I said, "I think I can feel my stomach muscles. Try letting go of me."

Deborah and Scott protested. "If we let go of you, you'll tip over."

"No, I can feel my back muscles too. Let go of me."

Deborah and Scott guardedly lifted their hands inches away from me, and I sat on my own.

Deborah started to cry. She said, "There is no physical explanation for what just happened. You've progressed so far in a single day."

Scott said, "I have chills. I've never seen anything like this in my medical career."

I looked at Megan and I started crying too. That was the first time I knew I could beat this. There was real hope. I might actually stand and walk again. I said, "Praise be to God." It was the first time I'd said those words in life and actually meant them.

Megan rushed over to hug me, and we cried into each other. It was awesome. It was powerful. A true miracle. Again, Paul's prayer had worked. We'd prayed to speed it up, and my recovery had defiantly sped up.

As soon as the therapy session ended, I had Megan call Paul and put the phone on speaker, "You'll never believe what happened!" I said.

He said, "Bet you I will believe! But please tell me."

# CHAPTER 26

# A Change of Scenery

Now that I could sit up, Dr. Berman ordered a "Cadillac" chair for me. Think of it as an electric recliner on wheels. They can tilt your legs up and your head up, and wheel you around.

Having the Cadillac chair allowed me to incline and decline more often throughout the day, with the added benefit of being mobile.

For me, it was a big deal to leave my room. I'd stared at the ceiling and those same four walls for nearly a month. My whole world was inside that box. With the exception of my ambulance ride from the ICU to Desert Canyon, I hadn't taken a whiff of outside air or even seen what the hospital looked like outside of my room.

With the Cadilac chair, I now had the option to get past my door, see the hallway outside, and learn the layout of the hospital. With this new device, my whole world changed and expanded. It's hard to describe the sense of adventure that can come from simply being able to wheel out of one room into the expansive world that lay beyond, even if that world was simply the building that housed me.

I also got to see other faces and began talking with fellow patients. I'm a social guy by nature, so it was great to have conversations with people that were, to one degree or another, going through what I was going through. I'd meet them in the hall, the dining room, and the therapy room. Wherever I ran into another patient, I'd try to strike up a conversation.

I quickly took note of what patients had the right mindset and those who didn't. Again, I was struck by how important effort and attitude are. Many patients were bitter, others had flat out given up. It made my heart break. I made an extra effort to be the hope to these people.

Since we understood more about each other's situations, fears, and pains than our loved ones and the staff, it seemed to me that we could encourage each other and learn from each other. I did my best to do my part, but they also needed to have the desire to not just survive, but to thrive.

With my new mobility, I wondered if they could wheel me outside. Desert Canyon has a beautiful courtyard with a little fountain in the middle. There were also flowers and trees. After weeks of looking at walls and ceiling tiles, this bit of nature was inspiring.

I remember that first morning when they wheeled me outside. The feeling of the sunshine was awesome. They put sunglasses on me and let me feel the clean, hot air. My hair was long and they hadn't washed it yet. So it was oily and slicked back, but this only intensified the warmth. Those moments in the sun's rays were the best thing ever. I lay there, soaking up as much of the sun as I could, breathing in as much air as my weak diaphragm could pull into my lungs.

And the smell of the desert air was like baking cookies to me. The heat pulling into my lungs felt delicious.

I was also sensitive to the sounds. The randomness of the splashing fountain was something you don't hear in man-made environments. There is a happiness to dancing water that hospitals don't have with all the beeps, motors, and routines.

I couldn't stay long, certainly not as long as I would have liked. I learned I had to be careful when I was outside. This was the beginning of June, which can be rather hot in Las Vegas. Within five minutes of being out in the sun, I began to get nauseated and dizzy.

I discovered that one of the considerations with spine injuries is your body doesn't respond correctly to hot or cold. My nurse, Scott Ryan, explained to me that normally, when you are hot, your body sends a signal to your brain that it is overheating, and the brain responds with the command to sweat. Unfortunately, my body's signals weren't getting through to my brain. Therefore, my brain would not tell my body to sweat. In turn, my core temperature would rise very quickly. So I had to be careful every time I went outside in the heat.

Trust me, if it meant being able to get a breath of fresh air, and the sight of some blue sky, it was worth it to take the necessary precautions. From that first day out of doors, we made it a point to go outside at least once a day.

# CHAPTER 27

# The Assurance of Insurance

Over the next week, there were several significant advances. Both my right and left feet were beginning to move, and I was able to bend my knees. Both hands had started to move, and I could bend both of my elbows slightly. With my eyes closed, I could tell where people were touching me. With each new sensation, we celebrated my healing.

Yes, my whole body was still completely numb, and every limb felt like it weighed 500 pounds. I still could not sit up by myself. It still took three people to get me upright on the side of the bed. And I couldn't roll from left to right, meaning I was still flat on my back most of the time. But I was making noticeable improvements, and for that, we were thankful.

Paul's words kept echoing in my head, "Well, let's pray to speed it up."

But all the progress came as a double-edged sword. The better I did, and the longer I stayed at the hospital, the closer we were to my insurance running out.

When we checked into Desert Canyon, we knew there would be a time when we'd have to check out. Desert Canyon was charging $1400 a day. According to my insurance policy, we had one month of in-patient rehab coverage. But as the days counted down, I still wasn't at the point where it was safe for me to be out of the hospital.

My mother, like most mothers, is a worrier. However, if there were a league for worriers, she'd be a professional. She started wringing her hands more as the days counted down. "What are we going to do if we have to take you home?" She would ask. "What are we going to do?"

"Mom, we'll work this out. But let's start praying on it." I tried to assure her.

She exclaimed, "How can you say that? We've got to *do* something."

I said, "I agree. We've got to make some phone calls." I learned that prayers can be answered, but often taking action is part of that answer.

One day, a member of my recovery committee, Karen Rogers, brought in an old fraternity brother of mine, Scott. I knew he was in Vegas, but we hadn't been in touch since we were in school together in the 1980s. All I remembered about Scott was his wry sense of humor.

Karen had run into Scott somewhere, and remembered that we knew each other in school. She told him about the accident, and he asked to see me.

When Karen brought Scott in, I said, "Hey, man, what's going on?"

He caught me up on his life, his business, and how he was the proud father of twins.

When I told him the story of my accident, I shared with him how I'd chosen to call my children when I thought I was going to die. His eyes welled up with tears. He said, "I can't imagine having to call my kids to say good bye."

When our time together was wrapping up, Scott, like so many others, asked, "What can I do to help?"

I don't know why I said what I said, perhaps it was because we were only days from the insurance running out and my mother's concerns were nagging in the back of my mind, but I said, jokingly, "If you know the president of my insurance company, you could give him a call because I need more time here."

He said, "Who's your insurance company?"

I told him.

He didn't say, "Let me make some phone calls," or anything like that. Instead, he just said, "OK," and we said our good byes.

Karen walked Scott to his car, and then came running back in, obviously excited.

I asked, "What?"

"Did Scott tell you he sits on the board of this hospital? And he owns the land that it's built on?"

"No, he didn't mention that."

"He's going to see what he can do to help!"

If I had known he was on the board, I'm not sure what I would have said to him, but I certainly wouldn't have thrown out the bit about the insurance company.

Meanwhile, Dr. Burman didn't want me to be discharged. He knew I needed more time. He began making appeals to the insurance company. He carefully documented all my needs, and how much I had progressed in such a short time. He argued that if I continued my intensive therapy, I would save the insurance company in the long-run.

For my part, I was working with lawyers, trying to figure out how I was going to finance my ongoing care. We talked with Social Security and Medicaid. They told me I'd have to stop working to get support.

I said, "So let me get this straight, in order for you to help me, I can't be working. But if I'm working and making a living, I don't qualify for any benefits?"

The answer was, "Yes."

It felt like they wanted me to be helpless and dependent. If I were working, I would be helping to fund the very programs that would be contributing to my care. It made no sense to me why I'd have to quit working.

Day 27 came and went. Then Day 28. And finally Day 29 came.

We started planning how we were going to handle things when I got home. The benefits administrator for the hospital was quickly preparing my discharge papers, making sure everything was in place the minute it was time to wheel me out of the room.

And yet, we still weren't sure how we would manage things. Yes, therapists could come to the house, but I was getting therapy seven days a week at the hospital. Plus, it took three to four people to transfer me, bathe me, lift me. Megan and my parents couldn't do that, nor were they available 24 hours a day.

Late in the day on Day 29, Dr. Burman walked into my room, shaking his head. "I don't know who you know, but you know the right people. I just got a call from the president of your insurance company. He assured me they will pay as long as you need to stay and as long as you keep making progress."

I was stunned. This was too amazing to be true. I said, "We are going to need that in writing. I don't want to stay under the pretense that they are going to pay and then 70 days later, I get the bill."

With all the miracles God had given me, I was still unwilling to trust the insurance company. We needed to protect ourselves. I had Megan write a memo stating that they acknowledge making the phone call to Dr. Burman and that they would pay the benefits as long as I continued to improve. Dr. Burman signed it and we faxed it to insurance company.

Sure enough, the offer was above board. They agreed they would cover me as long as I made progress. I smiled at Megan and said, "Well, now God is just showing off."

It's one thing for God to work with my physical body, it's quite another to compel a large, publicly-traded company to bend the rules and do something unprecedented for the likes of me.

It turned out Scott not only owned the land the hospital was built on and sat on the board of the hospital, he also sat on the same nonprofit board as the president of my insurance company. So when I jokingly asked, "Well, if you know the president of my insurance company...," he literally knew the president.

But I didn't know it was Scott who had done this for me. As soon as we had things settled that I would be staying, I got on the phone to ask who had authorized the care. It took a day and a half of calls before I found out that authorization had come from the president of the insurance company. I called him directly and asked what had compelled him to act on my behalf.

He told me, "Scott called and asked if there was anything I could do. We reviewed your policy and shifted some of your benefits around so you could pay for more inpatient therapy."

To this day, Scott downplays what he did. He doesn't want to talk about it, and he's uncomfortable with my thank-you letter and the free meals I've offered at our restaurants. He said, "All I did was make a call and ask if there was anything that could be done to help my buddy. That's all I did."

That isn't the end of the story with Scott. Three weeks later, Karen called. She was frantic, "Scott was bodysurfing in Laguna with his kids. He broke his neck."

My heart sank, "Oh God, don't tell me he's paralyzed."

She said, "He's moving."

I said, "Are you sure he's moving?"

"I don't have the details yet."

Later, Scott told me he was bodysurfing and dove under a wave. He hit a sand bar, and heard a loud crack. When the wave passed, he stood up. He turned his head to the right and to the left, then looked down. His arms and legs went numb for a second.

He thought, "This is bad."

He walked out of the ocean, drove himself to the hospital with his kids in the back seat. They took an X-ray and discovered that his C1 was broken in three places. One wrong move and he would be dead; not just paralyzed, but dead.

They did emergency surgery on him. He had to wear a halo for ten weeks. Fortunately, he suffered no paralysis nor lasting side effects.

He told me, "The first thing I thought of was 'Oh my God, I did what happened to Frost.'"

I told him, "When you helped me, you made a very large deposit in the karma bank. And you just made a sizeable withdrawal."

# CHAPTER 28

# An Introduction to Mr. Nielson

Now that I knew we had coverage for my care, and my recovery was accelerating, I had an increased sense of hope, and that hope helped suppress the ever present anxiety and worry. Of course, I was still uncomfortable and dealing with pain, and we knew that there would be setbacks, but our hope grew with each new victory.

With a renewed belief that God would continue to heal me, I began to look to the future. I knew that I would have the ability to support my family—I just needed to build my business. My injury was a physical one; God had preserved my voice and my brain. Most of my business day before the accident involved sitting at a desk and talking on the phone. I still had those abilities. The only skills I lacked were the ability to type and travel.

I remembered when I was in the ditch after the accident. I was thinking about the article I'd read about a casino executive,

Craig Nielson, who ran Ameristar Casinos as a quadriplegic. I was determined to find somebody who knew him and could share with me how he conducted his business.

After that day's therapy session, Meg and I were watching movies on a makeshift movie screen that consisted of a sheet draped over the armoire at the foot of my bed. We had a DVD player that could project onto the sheet.

The charge nurse, Rhonda Olson, popped her head in to say hi. It was after 10 PM and the hospital was quiet. She enjoyed chatting with Megan and me as she did her paperwork throughout the evening.

I asked her, "Hey, did you ever hear about Craig Nielson, the quad who ran his casino from bed?"

She grinned like the Cheshire Cat. "Yeah, I've heard of him."

I said, "So, did you know him?

"Yes, I worked for him for ten years before I came here."

I laughed. I was astonished. "Sit down, you and I have to talk."

I explained to her that I was thinking about how I was going to work in the future, and that I knew about Mr. Nielson, I just didn't know how he did it. So, I asked questions about how he conducted his daily life and how he held his meetings. I asked what she remembered most about him, and what she wished he'd done differently.

The answers were insightful. Mr. Nielson brought the office to him. He had Rhonda and another nurse by his bedside acting as both administrative assistants and caregivers. They rigged up a computer monitor that he could see from his bed as she typed on a laptop. He would dictate notes, look at floor plans, browse the Internet, review proposals, and so on all from his bed. Meanwhile, Rhonda acted as his hands.

When he needed to have meetings, he had his executives come into his room and sit around his bed. They would give their reports, he'd give them suggestions, and any notes that had to be taken would be written by Rhonda or the other assistant.

When he got tired, he'd excuse the people from his room. He had another room set up with food and beverages, a conference table, telephones, everything those people needed to keep working while he rested. When he awoke, he'd call everyone back in and they'd resume business.

Rhonda said what she admired most about Craig was that he was driven. But what she regretted most was for all his drive, he didn't try to recover physically after the accident. He accepted his physical condition and didn't think much about rehab.

I soaked all this information in while Megan took notes. I didn't have the resources that Craig Nielson had, but one thing I did have was the will to go through rehabilitation and the belief that I would be healed. I was not going to accept my physical condition. I was going to rebuild my body the same way I was going to rebuild my business.

People say it's a small world, but think about the chances that I would know about Mr. Nelson before I had my accident, that I would determine to follow in his footsteps once the accident happened, and finally, that one of two people who worked as Mr. Nelson's assistants was now taking care of me. It boggles the mind.

More important, what if I had never thought to ask Rhonda if she knew of Mr. Nelson? I would have lost the opportunity to gain insights into how to run a business when you're paralyzed. I also would not have had a plan for the path ahead.

God does work in mysterious ways.

# CHAPTER 29

# The Work Must Go On

I'd been at Desert Canyon for about three weeks when I heard that our proposal for the night club in Arizona had made it to the final round. We were competing with one other company. Now all they needed was a final presentation so they could compare the two companies and make the best decision for them. Of course, I thought we were the best decision, but we needed to prove it to them.

The last thing we wanted at this stage was to paint the picture that the guy running the company was in the hospital with a broken neck. So we made up an excuse about why I wasn't able to make the presentation in person. My partners, Brian Mangino and Jeff Marks, would travel to Arizona on my behalf and be present at the meeting. I would present the PowerPoint proposal we created via the phone.

Fortunately, Skype and Facetime weren't in general use yet, so the casino folks wouldn't expect to see me while I presented.

Instead, there were seven or eight people in their boardroom, listening to me on speakerphone as my partners advanced the PowerPoint slides for me.

On my side of the meeting, my Blackberry was on speaker and wedged in my neck brace. Megan worked through the PowerPoint so I knew where I was in the presentation. We did our best to make sure none of the sounds of the hospital made it across the telephone.

The only problem with this arrangement was I couldn't see the reactions of the principles at the meeting. I couldn't judge if they were understanding me, or how they felt about what I was presenting. I couldn't even tell if they were listening.

Then again, they couldn't see that I was lying flat in a bed, my head held immobile with a neck brace, looking out of the corner of my eyes at the laptop as Megan clicked the return key.

Perhaps the most difficult part of the presentation is that I needed to sound like I was able bodied and seated at an executive's desk. It's difficult to project your voice when you're on your back and your head is level with your chest. Having a phone propped against a brace and on speaker was not the best audio approach to a phone presentation. Worse, my diaphragm was weak from being paralyzed and in little use since the accident. It took everything I had to focus on the presentation while projecting my voice, adding depth and confidence that I didn't feel.

Given the limitations, I thought the presentation went well. It wasn't ideal, but Megan agreed that I had made a good argument as to why we were the better choice. Now all we could do was wait to hear from the client.

The following days were nerve-wracking. Megan watched my phone throughout the day, ready to prepare me to answer it as soon as an Arizona number appeared on the screen. When it stayed silent, we fretted. When it rang, she jumped to see the number. When it wasn't them, she'd disappointedly tell me who it was, or simply shake her head in resignation.

Then, finally, the screen showed the Arizona number. Megan beamed as she positioned my phone into my neck brace. I had a surge of elation and dread as she pushed the receive button. "Hello. This is Scott Frost."

I looked into Megan's eyes while they explained to me that they had gone with the other company.

I asked why.

The casino owner said, "The other guy is from Arizona, and has some experience here. I think they might be a better option for us."

My heart sank. Everything we'd done, all the effort, creativity, long hours, and now this. What if I had been able to attend the meeting in person? What if I hadn't gone motorcycle riding that day? Not only was my family now in peril, but so were the many people working with me. So many people were relying on this contract. If I had simply jumped off the bike, or tucked my head, or even rested the bike on the floor of the retention basin, we wouldn't be in the place. I would have been able to travel to Arizona and given the best possible presentation ever. In general, when people meet me, hear what I have to say, they respect me and understand me. Now I was reduced to making phone calls from my bed, not even able to hold the phone to my ear.

I've learned not to burn bridges, so I thanked the casino representative for the opportunity to bid on the project, and asked him to let us know if anything changed.

I was defeated. It was in that emotional space that I called my partners and told them the news They were incredulous and bummed out. They affirmed that it had been a good idea that the casino didn't know about my accident and that I was in a rehab hospital. Beyond that, there wasn't much else we could have done differently.

Instead of dwelling on our disappointment, we needed to focus on our other project, a Mexican restaurant in the Mandalay Bay Resort and Casino called Hussong's Cantina.

As a demonstration of our new focus and resolve, Jeff and I immediately called Mandalay Bay to resume lease negotiations.

Because Mandalay Bay is in Las Vegas, and news of my accident traveled fast, our landlord, Brian Robison, was acutely aware of my condition. It didn't appear to affect the negotiations one way or the other; they simply wanted to get a lease signed.

Jeff worked diligently on the lease revisions throughout the week, as we batted the ball back and forth with Mandalay Bay.

On that Friday, we wrapped up the final details on the phone. Jeff affixed my digital signature that we had prior to my accident and faxed the lease agreement over. It was game on.

I was ecstatic and so thankful that I could still participate in life and pursue my career.

Now that we had a lease agreement, it was time to ramp up the project. The next hurtle was paying for the project. Jeff is the yin to my yang. I tend to be paranoid and aggressive, and he tends to be trusting and passive, which is odd because he is a lawyer. Together we make a good team, balancing each other out.

I got on the phone with some of our early investors to make sure everyone was on board. We needed to solidify the financial commitments and set things in motion. The investors anticipated that we would get the lease, so it wasn't like I was cold-calling them. All I needed to do was let them know that we had, indeed, gotten the lease, and ask for their financial commitment as we moved into the next stage.

The people I was talking with were local, and they all knew my situation. I was nervous that they would shy away from their investment because of my accident. From their perspective, I might be bed-ridden the rest of my life. They were not aware of the small, almost daily, miracles that were happening.

Of the handful of investors I spoke with, only one dropped out. He said, "Scott, I had faith in you, but now that you are in the position you are in, I am out."

My mouth went dry when he said those words. I felt pain in my heart. I was scared that we were not going to be able to raise the rest of the money. We were well short of the investment needed, and if my close business associates didn't have faith in me and my company, how would we raise the rest of the money?

I called Jeff to let him know what the investor had said. Jeff's reply was, "I'll work on it."

Jeff began a conversation with his uncle who runs the CPA firm Rose, Snyder & Jacobs. Together they created an offer we could syndicate through them.

In a matter of days, I received a call from Jeff, "I think we've got the money raised."

"Praise God!" I thought, "We were going to have a restaurant. I will be able to support my family!" All we had to do now was open the restaurant. And we had a few short months to pull it off.

If I weren't helpless, dependent on others for the very basics of life, I would have been thrilled with the challenge. I would have spent long hours at the office and on-site, overseeing all the details, making sure every detail was addressed, and anticipating even the slightest hick-up. Instead, I was stuck in a hospital with hours of therapy and long, deep naps. I was filled with trepidation. How could I oversee this project on top of all my daily struggles?

I thought back through everything that had happened to this point. What is the opposite of what I feared? God had brought me this far; he was going to take me the rest of the way. He would not have put me in this position if He wasn't going to continue to provide.

Declaring my belief that God would continue to work miracles, I decided to set another audacious goal. I turned to Megan and said, "I'm going to walk through the front door of Hussong's Cantina at the grand opening."

I said that at a time when I couldn't even stand or move my legs, but the audacious goal became a new battle cry. I could picture in my mind how amazing it would be for everyone to see me walking. Of course, at that point, I couldn't even visualize what the restaurant would like, where the bar would be in relationship to the hallway. I remembered the space that existed the last time I had toured the property before the accident, but that was it. So I focused on the faces of my friends, family, and business associates who I was sure would be at the grand opening. I saw the looks on their faces as I strolled into the restaurant on my own two feet.

At that point, we had no idea how long I was going to be in the hospital. We couldn't delay business meetings until I was able to formally visit an office. Our time was short, so we had to move forward quickly.

I asked if there was a conference room at the hospital.

They said, "What for?"

I said, "We're building a restaurant at Mandalay Bay. I need to have a place for meetings."

They shook their heads. "Who are you?"

"I'm just trying to make a living."

They said, reluctantly, "Yes, there is a conference room."

We solicited proposals from several local architects. Then we stacked their presentations so we could get through them all in one afternoon. Each architect had one hour. It was going to be physically exhausting for me to get through them all, but I didn't see an alternative.

I did physical therapy in the morning. Then I took a nap. When Megan woke me, the hospital staff cleaned me up as best they could without a shower or shampoo. They did shave my face. I asked to have a dress shirt and tie to look at least a little bit professional, but I had to have sweat pants on, and since I would be in my Cadillac chair, my sweats would be more visible than my shirt. It was the best we could do.

Out of vanity perhaps, but probably more out of concern for scaring the presenters, I took off my neck brace.

As I was being wheeled to the conference room, I went past Dr. Burman. He looked at me but kept going. It had only been about four weeks since the accident, and I was supposed to wear the brace for ten weeks. I knew this, so I was being careful not to move my head. Still, I cringed as we passed, the same way you might when you're speeding past a police car. You look in your rearview mirror, relieved when they don't come after you. I was relieved when Dr. Burman didn't say anything.

We began at noon and went straight through until 3:00 PM. I can imagine what the architects were thinking when they pulled up to the hospital and were ushered into the conference room. Worse, at the head of the conference table was this big man propped into a huge Cadillac chair with sweatpants on and a shirt that didn't quite cover his scars. He couldn't move much, and was keeping his head oddly still.

I started the presentation with, "Thank you for coming to my new office. I know these are unusual circumstances..."

To their credit, the presenters were cordial, dealing with the sight of me, skin and bones with a big, gnarly scar on my neck, plus the surroundings and my equipment. They did their dog-and-pony shows professionally, and I'd ask a few questions while Megan took notes.

Everything went well. I'm sure the different surroundings and the position of their audience put extra pressure on the presenters. I'm also sure they wondered how this guy would ever open and run a restaurant in a major casino. I doubt any of them put much stock into the possibility that their proposal would eventually become a renowned Las Vegas restaurant.

I made it through all the presentations with my energy level intact. We didn't even rush the last person out of the hospital. They had as much time and consideration as the first one.

When they left, Megan wheeled me back to my room so we could put the neck brace back on. Then we removed my tie and dress shirt, and prepared for afternoon therapy.

I was dressed as my usual patient self when Dr. Burman came into my room. Evidently I hadn't dodged the speeding ticket after all. He said, in his usual quiet manner, "What are you doing?"

"I had a couple of meetings today." I said, half defensively, half apologetically.

He said, "Do you want to be completely paralyzed for the rest of your life? If you moved the wrong way and severed your spine, you would be completely paralyzed with no hope of recovery. Or you could die.

He paused, hoping his words would set in, "Do not take your neck brace off again."

I had never seen Dr. Burman upset. I knew this was his version of blowing up at me. I took his warning seriously. Dr. Burman is a quiet man. He didn't like what he saw, and he let me know how frustrated he was with me in the sternest way he knew how.

I let him know that I heard his warning.

The following Monday, the casino in Arizona called back. We almost missed the call. When Megan looked at the phone, she gave a little start. We hadn't expected to see their phone number on the screen again. She quickly positioned the phone under my neck brace.

When she nodded that she had answered the call, I said, "This is Scott Frost."

The casino representative identified himself and then got straight to the point, "We aren't going to work with the other guy. If you want to open the club, you can have the contract."

I was dumbstruck. I had mentally set aside the disappointment and was focusing on the restaurant. Now I was being given the nightclub opportunity as well.

I paused before answering, "Of course. We'd be happy to take it."

He said, "Can you please forward a proposal to me that is on your terms."

They were in a tight spot. They were getting ready to open their casino in less than four months and the night club was a big part of the grand opening. And they didn't have an operator lined up. So I set the terms in our favor. Now that we had the restaurant moving forward, we would need extra resources to be able to open their club while continuing to get the restaurant up and ready for launch.

Lying in my hospital bed that afternoon, I thought to myself, "This is crazy. How can we take on two projects at the same time while I'm still in the hospital?"

Deborah Howell's words echoed in my head, "Effort and attitude."

The good news was that all the extra work would keep my mind off of my situation and would reinforce the philosophy that I'm the same guy from the shoulders up. I can contribute and be productive even though I'm paralyzed. I have a future. The pain I was enduring would help me succeed later.

Instead of focusing on the "how," I began to trust that God would put the people and resources that we needed into place. All I had to do was be ready. I was excited to see how this adventure would play out.

# CHAPTER 30

# Standing Tall

Another week past, and I was finally able to begin to tolerate sitting up for longer periods of time. Now we could really get to work on physical therapy.

First, I'd have to learn to stabilize myself with my own hands and body while sitting up in the therapy center. The problem was I didn't have the arm strength, nor did my hands work well. I had these non-functioning "gorilla" hands. When I'd flex my wrist backward, my fingers would pull in like a gorilla walking on his knuckles.

They wanted me to put my hands flat, pressing them down on either side of me. In theory, I should have enough leverage to scoot down the bed like this. But my hands weren't right, and my arms not coordinated enough. Also, my core was still weak. But the more I struggled, the better I got, and the more functional my hands became.

Just as I was getting the hang of scooting down my bed, they put what they called a "slide board" between my bed and my wheelchair. They maneuvered me so my butt was on the board. The idea was to use my hands and core to scoot down the board in order to transfer from the bed to the wheelchair.

The problem was I was unable to scoot. The technique involves leaning forward, putting your nose past your toes to make your butt lighter. Then you push down with your hands and shift your butt sideways along the board. With weak arms and no way to grab on to something should I lean too far forward, it felt like I was going to fall all the way over, planting my face on the ground. So not only did I have physical limitations, I also had the mental limitation of fear of falling on my face.

So the simple task of moving my butt along a board was both difficult and scary. I remember yelling at Deborah "I'd rather just stand up and pivot and sit in the chair."

She said, "It doesn't work that way. You want to get from A to C, and this B."

I exclaimed, "Forget B. I want to go to C."

She challenged me, "Then you'd better learn to stand up!"

There was nothing I wanted to do more than stand up, but I barely had function of my arms and a little feeling in my feet. I was a long way from standing.

When I first checked into Dessert Canyon, I told the medical staff that I didn't want a day off. This meant I did therapy on the weekends as well. It also meant I'd see different therapists on Saturday and Sundays.

These weekend sessions may not have been as intense as during the week, but my body still got a good workout.

Damon Elliot was my weekend therapist. He was built like a wrestler. In fact, he was training in Mixed Martial Arts as he completed his physical therapy degree. Despite how menacing he looked, he was a really mellow guy.

Damon came from a different school of thought when it came to physical therapy. The techniques on which he was trained didn't involve machines; it was all about biomechanics. This meant that the therapist would use leverage, physics, and sheer strength to take the place of machines.

One Sunday, he was wheeling me down the hall when I asked, "What are we going to work on today?"

He said, "I'm going to stand you up."

"How are you going to do that?"

He said, "Don't worry. I'll show you."

When we got to the physical therapy room, he forced me to struggle with the slide board again to get onto the therapy table. Then he explained, "I'm going to put my shoulder into your chest and put your arms over my head like I'm tackling you. Then I'm going to put my knees against your knees. I'm going to put my arms around the small of your back. I'll pull your hips forward while bracing your knees and pushing my shoulder into your chest. Like that, we are going to stand you up."

I nodded, apprehensive.

It took a few seconds to get into position. Then Damon said, "Ready?"

Tentatively, I answered, "Yes."

He said, "I want you to concentrate on pushing your hips forward. Brace your knees. We are going to stand you up. One. Two. Three."

It was like butter. In one smooth motion I was standing. Of course, he was hugging me and taking most of my weight, but I was tall again. I was upright and looking over his head at the room beyond. It put a smile on my face. If it only took one person to make me stand, there was hope that I could do it by myself someday.

Damon slowly let me back down. I began to laugh. "You made that look easy."

He just smiled and said, "Ready to do it again?"

We repeated the maneuver two more times. As much as I was enjoying it, three times was all I could take.

By the time Damon got me back to my room, I was shot. I fell quickly into a "power coma." It was funny how exhausting it could be to have someone lift and hug me into a standing position.

The gift that Damon gave me was a feeling of being tall again. I wasn't a victim destined to lay flat on my back the rest of my life. I knew what it would feel like to again be standing tall.

Before Deborah arrived the next morning, the nurses got me dressed as usual, only this time they put shoes on me. It looked odd to be laying in bed with shoes on, waiting for therapy.

When Deborah arrived, she said, "Okay, get your feet over the edge of the bed."

I looked at her in disbelief, "I can't do that."

She said, "I want you to try."

To this day, it's not an easy maneuver. Back then, it was a 15-minute process. I had to squirm to move my right foot a half inch, and labor to get my left foot to follow. I struggled and struggled. But even with all the effort, I'd only moved my feet about five inches toward the edge.

Mercifully, she helped me, pulling my feet over. Scott got behind me, lifting me to a seated position. When I swayed, fear shot through me. I didn't have control of my body. I could fall to the left or right or forward. Yes, Deborah and Scott were there to grab me, but I still felt vulnerable.

Deborah steadied me with a hand on my shoulder and said, "I heard you stood up yesterday."

I smiled.

She said, "I have a machine that will help you do that more often."

That sounded like a good thing until I saw the machine. It looked like something from Medieval times. It was called a "sit-stand machine." It involved a harness underneath the back of my thighs and across my torso. Once standing there was a table that surrounded my upper body for my arms to rest on. The idea was that my shoulders would bear some of my weight by pressing my arms onto the surrounding table. The problem was I could not stand and my shoulders weren't very strong.

It took Deborah and the team over ten minutes just to get me in the thing.

When they finally pulled on all the straps, Deborah asked if I was ready.

I wasn't sure how this machine was going to work. The belt around my torso started to pull me up. My butt was in one position, but the straps were pulling my shoulders up to the point it felt like they were going to snap my lower back.

I screamed, "Stop! Stop! Stop!"

Deborah said, "Hold on." And then she worked on the machine for a bit. When she was satisfied she'd fixed things, she said, "Trust me. We are going to go a little slower this time. I think we have it in the right spot."

It started to pull, but then it stopped. The straps under my legs started to push my hips forward.

She said, "You've got to push those legs. I know you've got some muscle coming back. Lean forward, the harness has you. When you get to an upright position, we are going to pull your arms up."

Slowly the machine pulled me into a standing position. Finally they had me upright. I felt 6'7" again.

My elation was fleeting because this process was excruciating. My shoulders were trying to take some weight, my lower back was stretching, my legs were not strong enough to hold my body up, and the harness was pulling on the inside of my crotch.

The point of the torture was to teach my brain what it was like to stand up.

In a few short weeks, Deborah had moved me from the tilt-table, which was one form of torture, to this new machine, which was a whole new form of torture, preparing me to stand on my own. The sit-stand machine was the bane of my existence for a solid week. I hated it because it hurt and it was difficult.

I only survived because Deborah explained, "It's all about the synapses in your brain. Your brain is firing signals, but only some are getting through. We've got to keep firing the signals that it is okay to stand upright."

Physical therapy was such an involved process. I had no idea how intricately the body processes are and how dependent each part is upon the others. I wish that before the accident, I had appreciated how easily my body moved.

# CHAPTER 31

# First Steps

How could I ever hope of walking into Hussong's Cantina when it opened? I'd stood up, sort of, but taking actual steps was a pipe dream. While standing was cool, I needed Damon or the machine to get me there and hold me there. I couldn't move my feet; instead, they were barely holding me in place. I was a long way from shifting my weight to one foot and lifting the other.

Deborah assured me she had another machine for that; it was called the gait walker.

Imagine a big metal doorway on wheels. It has a harness that hooks to the top of the "doorway." The harness goes between your legs, around your chest, and over your shoulders. The shoulder straps then hook onto the cross bar overhead. There's a handle on the side to crank up the hooks so the straps bear your weight.

Since the machine is on wheels, two people stand on either side to first of all hold the machine in place and then to move it forward as I began to take steps. With most of my weight off my feet, I could focus on lifting one foot high enough to swing it forward with a therapist guiding the foot.

The first time, it took about 20 minutes to get all hooked up. But then we found out I was too tall for the machine. My head was hitting the top of the "doorway." By shortening the shoulder straps, they got my body just where it needed to be.

Once I was in, we were ready to take my first steps. I was excited but nervous. I stared with my right foot, willing my knee to lift my foot off the ground. Nothing happened.

"Come on," I thought. "Come on. All I need is one inch. Push.

Still nothing happened. I took a deep breath. Looked up. I said, "One step for mankind. One giant leap...," and tried again.

Suddenly, my right foot shifted forward three inches. Megan put her hands to her face. I looked at her as if I'd just performed a magic trick.

Now it was time to move my left leg. My left foot was slightly behind me, so when I pushed down on my right leg and tried to move my left forward, my left knee locked backwards. As hard as I tried to get my knee to bend forward and lift my left foot, it simply wouldn't move.

One of the therapists, Ed Hladek, yelled, "Reset! Breathe. Relax. Move your right foot forward more. Take a bigger step this time."

I did what he said. Took a breath. Concentrated again on my right foot. Ed reached for it. I told him to let go. With all my might, I moved my right foot forward again, four inches. This bigger step made it easier for my left knee to bend the correct way.

Leaning forward and concentrating on lifting my left heel, I struggled to slide my left foot forward. Finally, Ed assisted my left foot and moved it past my right. I reluctantly accepted the help. It moved the gait walker forward another foot.

And now it was time to try the right foot again. The process was grueling. I had to break everything down and do it by the numbers. Push up. Lean forward. Keep nose over toes. Shift weight. Pull the other knee. Drag the foot forward. Pause. And repeat on the other side. We would later nickname it, "Frankenstein walking."

Unless you are paralyzed, you have no idea the amount of physical effort it takes to slide your foot a couple of inches. I could look at my leg, will it to move, and nothing happened. It was crazy how maddening this process was. Eventually, something would kick in and the foot would move.

That first day, with everybody's help, we went almost eight feet. Meg stood in front of me with a video camera. I watched her slowly step backward as I made progress. I was thinking, "It's working. This is going to happen."

Everyone could see how much effort I was exerting, and the connection between Meg and me. They saw her dedication and how strong she was. Looking in her eyes, as I shuffled along, she was my inspiration.

Eventually, of course, my body collapsed in sheer exhaustion. But I had walked, actually walked. Yes, it took a lot of assistance, but these feet of mine had moved forward. I'd taken steps! All that was left was doing it better and more easily. Soon, I'd be walking on my own.

# CHAPTER 32

# Clean

One of the most simple things that we take for granted is being clean. It was almost six weeks after my accident, and I hadn't taken a real bath.

I kept asking the nurses, "When do I get to take a bath? When can you shampoo my head? When can I have actual hot water on my body?"

It turned out Dr. Burman hadn't cleared me for this activity because they needed to take my neck brace off during the showering process. I swear, Dr. Burman was punishing me for the stunt I had pulled when I took my neck brace off to have the meetings.

Finally, they said, "We can do it tonight."

I was excited like a kid waiting for Christmas. And like that kid, I had to wait.

The hospital was full of elderly patients who seemingly all wanted to go to bed at the same time, between 7:00 and 9:00

PM. Before that could happen, they had to eat, take their meds, and deal with whatever was bothering them before the lights went out. The nurses ran around hectically during those few hours, trying to keep everyone happy and get them to sleep.

During the evening rush, I would purposefully stay quiet and try not to be needy. Why? Because after 9:00, I had the nursing staff all to myself.

Once the last person was comfortable and their lights dimmed, a hush settled over the hospital.

That's how it was the night I got my first bath. It was close to 10:00 PM, and I lay there wondering how they were going to get this 6'7" man, who now weighed a mere 220 pounds (down from my pre-accident weight of 275), and can't move a muscle, into the bath.

I heard something rolling down the hall toward my room. I strained my eyes toward the door. In rolled a gurney made out of PVC pipe so it can be considered waterproof. There was a railing on the sides, but otherwise, it didn't look like a secure form of transportation.

They lifted my bed to the same height as the "shower" gurney. But because of the railing, they had to lift me up and over and back down onto the gurney. Sure it was only four inches up and a few inches over, but it was rather high for lifting this big body.

Worse, the gurney was made for someone who was shorter than six foot. With my neck brace, they couldn't have my head hanging over one end, so my feet were going to dangle over the other.

One person got on each corner of my sheet, and one positioned himself underneath. On three, they all lifted me up and over the PVC pipping. They carefully maneuvered my head inside the gurney, but now my Achilles tendons on both legs were resting on the four inch railing at the end. And it hurt. I was thankful that I could feel the sensation, but it was uncomfortable nonetheless. They couldn't bend my legs and fit my feet inside because I couldn't control my legs. They'd flop to the left or right, or spread, putting strain on my painful right hip. The best they could do was put a pillow underneath my knees and ankles to pad the railing.

Once that process was completed, they wheeled me into a bathroom where there was a sink and a big shower stall. When I saw it, I christened it "The Human Car Wash." The shower stall wasn't big enough to roll the whole bed in, but the big shower head was connected to a hose, so they could spray me down like a car.

They removed the sheet from above me and then gingerly removed my neck brace, leaving me totally naked for the first time since before the accident.

Now that I was ready, they began spraying me down. The first time I felt hot water on my head, it was like heaven. Now when I watch westerns, I know how those old-timers felt when they came into town and had a bath.

I felt the water penetrating all the grease in my hair, reaching my scalp. As the grime washed away, a feeling of lightness took its place.

What was weird was I could only feel the heat of the water from my chest up. I knew the rest of my body was getting wet, I could feel the pressure from the spray, and there were spots of hot on my body, but for the most part I couldn't tell that the rest of my body was getting washed.

You can't be modest when you're paralyzed. I was lying there, buck naked, with four nurses washing me. I joked, "There's guys who pay a lot of money for this kind of treatment in Las Vegas." Then I thought about it. "Wait a minute, I *am* paying a lot of money."

Everyone laughed.

They rolled me to the left to clean my backside, and then onto my right to make sure all of me was clean.

When they were done, they put the neck brace back on before towelling me off. The brace had gotten a little soggy, but it was worth the opportunity to feel clean.

When I was as dry as possible, they then rolled me back and forth to get a new sheet under me. Then they wheeled me back to my room where they reversed the earlier process, lifting me up and over the PVC railing and back into bed.

It felt like a whole new bed now that I was clean. In fact, I felt like a new person in my new bed. For all the work, it was worth it. I can't describe how good it felt to have the grime off my body, to feel the lightness of clean hair, to have had warm water wash over me.

It took five people at least an hour to get me showered, so I didn't get a bath very often, but when I did, I counted it as one of my best blessings.

# CHAPTER 33

# The Walk

I was progressing with the gait walker. I was now able to do 20 foot "laps" across the room. But it wasn't enough to satisfy Deborah. She had another contraption in mind for me.

Her next machine was the platform walker. This machine looks like a regular walker with two poles on either side. Atop these poles are little platforms for my elbows to rest on. It looked like one of those futuristic jet packs strapped to a walker.

Even though I couldn't move my arms very well, I could use my shoulder muscles and some of my chest muscles to help me stay upright.

It took three people to get me into the walker, but once I was there, they could step away, and for the first time I was fully standing with no one holding on to me. It was a real sense of freedom.

In the platform walker, I had one person behind me to make sure I didn't fall backwards, one person monitoring the walker itself, and one person kneeling in front of me, helping guide my feet forward.

I was having to learn to walk all over again. Sometimes I would "scissor step," where one foot would cross over the other foot. My left knee was still locking and my toes were dragging. So each step was a monumental effort.

Making matters worse, I couldn't feel where my feet were. I had to look down at them. I couldn't look ahead, like most people, and trust that my feet were moving. While I could feel pressure on the soles, walking was like being in huge snowboots. All I could feel was the movement of my legs. That was it. I didn't know if my heel was hitting the ground or even if my foot was straight.

It's hard to describe the sensation where you are trying with all your might to move something, and it won't move. It's the most confounding sensation to stare at your foot, arm, or even finger, and not have it move. The funny part is that it can be exhausting watching it not move. I'd be holding my breath, trying to will the body part to move and nothing would happen. The therapists would see me struggling and tell me to breathe. Holding my breath wasn't helping me.

There was a hallway right outside the gymnasium. It was wide enough that people could get around me as I struggled forward. Deborah would wheel me into the hallway in my wheelchair and the staff would pull me up into the platform walker and strap my forearms onto the platform with my hands on the handles.

My rehab team learned quickly that the way to motivate me was to measure my progress and then challenge me to beat my progress the previous day. They learned that quantifying things gave me targets to shoot for.

Having goals was key to my recovery. Once I got into the platform walker and started to take some steps, progress was not only easier to measure, but also more dramatic.

That first day, I went about eight feet. The second day, I beat eight feet and went for 12 feet. The next day it was 14 feet and 8 inches.

My right leg was weaker from all the knee surgeries I've had in the past. So I would take "big" steps moving my right leg forward, then take a shorter step with my left because my right leg could only stay locked for a short time. The challenge we had with my left leg, which was my "good knee," was that as it bore all the weight, it would hyper-extend. They were concerned that I would tear a ligament.

To help me out, they got me a Bledsoe brace, which was a thigh to ankle brace. It has a dial on the side with a lock so it couldn't go past a certain degree. This kept my left knee from hyper-extending.

So I had a sleeve on my right knee, a Bledsoe brace on my left knee, a belt around my waist so people could hold on to me, and I was standing in a platform walker. It didn't look like I was walking, but I was.

The hallway was probably 50 or 60 feet long, and then it took a right turn. From there, it was another 200 feet to the nurses' station. At first, I would walk 10 to 12 feet, and they'd put me in the wheelchair to rest. Then I'd get back in the walker and do another 10 to 12 feet. Then rest again.

Soon I could make it to the corner without a rest. When I turned the corner and saw the nurses' station, it seemed like such a long way away. But we were progressing toward it.

One morning, after I'd warmed up, I said, "Hey, we're going to the nurses' station today." Once again, setting an audacious goal.

Scott Ryan said, "If you make it to the nurses' station, I'll give you a bath myself."

The nurses' station was three times further than I'd ever gone before. But I was feeling good.

I began walking, moving past the mark we'd reached the day before, 72 feet. Eyeballing the nurses' station, I just kept on truckin'. It was strange, I felt strong. Something was telling me that I could do it.

When I was a third of the way down the hallway, they said, "Scott, you need to slow down. You need to sit and rest."

"I'm feeling fine." I said, gritting my teeth. I was tired, but the excitement of reaching the nurses station had taken over.

At this point in the hall, I was now passing by other patients' rooms. I was seeing how others lived in the hospital. This was also the first time many of the patients had seen me standing up and walking. One lady exclaimed, "Gosh, you're tall."

People in other rooms offered encouragement, saying things like, "You're doing great. Keep going!"

Finally, I was 30 feet from the nurses' station. Word had travelled about what was going on. A crowd gathered. The nurses were all there, cheering me on. My walking became sloppy. I scissor-stepped. When I did, we'd stop, back up and reset my feet. Then I'd dragged my toes.

With all my struggles, Deborah started worrying. She didn't want me to collapse or fall. She offered to sit me down in the wheelchair.

I refused. "We are almost there. We are going to do this. Don't worry."

I was five feet away. Then four. Then three.

When the wheels of the platform walker hit the side of the nurses' station, people were clapping and crying. I was laughing with the joy of accomplishment. Who could have guessed I would get this far this quickly?

They pulled the wheelchair up behind me, and I collapsed into it. I was dripping with sweat. I had made it!

That achievement inspired everybody. All of the nurses and some of the patients had seen me when I first came to Desert Canyon. They knew how far I had come. My progress bore witness to the possibility of miracles and how God enables us to accomplish more than we think is physically possible. My feat had touched everyone in the building.

The walk showed that I wouldn't be limited to a chair the rest of my life. I would be able to walk, maybe not without assistance, but I would be walking. All of the little miracles were coming together to create a bigger, more dramatic, one.

I felt like I had won a championship game. When I got back to my room, I called my parents to tell them about the accomplishment. And then I slept for two and half hours.

# CHAPTER 34

# Father's Day

Besides those few hours in ICU before my surgery, I hadn't seen my children since the afternoon before the accident. Yes, we were trying to protect them. I wanted to be in as good as shape as possible before they visited me. They'd already been shocked by the tubes and my beat up body when I was in ICU, now I wanted them to see a more healed me.

There were also logistical problems. The kids were now living with their mother in Boulder City, which was a long way from my hospital. And while Taylor was 16, she wasn't driving yet, and their mother worked full-time. Getting them to see me when my schedule allowed for visitors was difficult.

Plus, I think all of us were unsure of what it would be like to reconnect in person. I was working hard to become physically more presentable, and I know the kids were struggling with their new reality of a paralyzed father. Also, their mother wanted their lives to be a normal as possible.

A day would pass, and I'd think I still wasn't where I wanted to be when the kids saw me for the first time. I was just now standing and walking a bit, but I still had all this equipment around me. Then, when I'd stumble or struggle in therapy, I'd think I wasn't ready to present myself to my kids. What would they think of a weak and awkward father?

I wanted to assure my children that I was the same dad from the shoulders up, but after an intensive physical therapy session, I didn't always feel that way. I'm sure if I looked even deeper, I'd acknowledge that I was wracked with guilt about how my injuries would affect the rest of their lives.

My daughter's nickname for me is "Daddy Man." She meant that I was like a superhero to her. When she was a child, I was larger than life. She had the belief that, like a superhero, I could accomplish anything. If she needed something fixed or needed help, I'd be there.

What kind of a superhero could I be helpless in a bed? Now they'd have to be picking up after me. They'd have to be the caregivers for their dad. And at 14 and 16, they weren't at the stages in life where they should be worrying about the physical limitations of their father. I could only imagine how tough it was for them.

Again, no one prepares you for this. There isn't a book that tells you the best way to prepare children whose parents are now paralyzed. I'm not sure we did the right thing when it came to the kids. I have talked with them extensively since, and it doesn't sound like the end results would have been better or worse if we'd done thing differently. For all of us, this time of upheaval was intense, but the kids, ultimately, have suffered from not having a physically strong father.

But as Father's Day approached, it made sense to arrange a time for the kids to see me. After all, I was making significant progress and I had audacious goals of walking. Besides, my physical limitations would be their new normal.

Usually, Father's Day for us was an active weekend. We'd escape the heat of Las Vegas for an adventure. But now, who knew what Father's Day would be like next year or the year after?

When the day arrived, I was more excited then I'd been in a long time. Just to see Christian and Taylor again would mean the world to me. I ached to look upon them, to feel their touch.

I knew instinctively when they entered the hospital. I knew the steps I heard were theirs. I became nervous as I heard them approaching my room. The staff had cleaned me up and dressed me as best they could with a big neck brace getting in the way and feet and legs that don't go easily into shoes and pants.

Taylor was first in the room. I cranked my eyes sideways to witness her coming. Quickly, she moved to stand in front of me, holding up a big poster. On bright orange posterboard, she'd placed big words across the top saying, "Daddy Man can do anything." The D was in the shape of the Superman logo.

Under that title, Taylor had written my favorite lines from movies and songs. There were also the logos from my favorite sports teams and pictures of important times in our lives.

My eyes teared up. It was the perfect present. Inspirational and motivational. We hung the poster in my line of sight. And it followed me home at the end of my hospital stay. For the next year and a half, that poster hung where I could see it.

Christian was a little more hesitant, lagging behind his sister. He smiled tentatively, staying on the edge of my sight line. I could tell he was scared. In some ways, I think it was harder on him to see me this way.

Trying my best to show off, I shuffled my feet toward the edge of the bed. The head nurse and Megan swung my feet over the edge and helped me sit up. They placed the platform walker in front of me, and Megan and Scott Ryan helped me stand up. I was tall again for the kids, looming large above the platform walker.

The kids looked up at me and smiled. One at a time, they maneuvered their way under my arms, positioning themselves between me and the platform walker. For the first time in weeks, I felt first my daughter's arms around me, and then my son's.

I had had kisses since the accident, and people had stroked my head and arms, but I had not stood up and had someone wrap their arms around me. I didn't realize how much I missed being hugged until that moment, and my kids were the ones who delivered the good feelings to me. It was the best feeling in the world.

Even now, I don't get hugged a lot because I'm in my chair most of the time. Before the accident, I was a hugger. I hugged pretty much everyone. I miss how it feels to be close to someone, the tactile comfort that comes from feeling them wrap their arms around you.

My daughter is tall, but my son was shorter at the time. He moved in for his turn to hug me. When he did, I heard him whisper, "God, I miss this."

I don't think he knew I heard him, or even if he realized he said it aloud, but it felt so good to know his feelings. I realized then how much I missed my kids. I wished I could hug them back like they were hugging me. Instead, all I could do was accept their love, lightly draping my arms around them.

Because my accident had been covered on the news, my children had a lot of support. Their peers and teachers knew the situation. Both kids had some struggles academically, as you would expect with all that was going on in their lives, but with the extra help and attention, they ended up doing all right. I'm proud of how they handled the situation. They never quit or got angry about the unfairness of what had happened to me. They are survivors, just like their dad.

Christian slipped back from underneath my arms. It was time to sit back down. Scott and Megan swung my legs back around so I could be comfortable in bed.

I asked the kids how they were doing. After the initial round of small talk about school, what they were involved with after school, and how they were holding up, they began to relax. I joked with them, trying to reassure them that inside, I was still the dad they knew and loved. But I noticed them stealing glances at my body, neck brace, and the room. They did their best to pretend this was a normal situation, but it wasn't.

The visit didn't last long enough. I was tired from therapy that day, and I knew that they still felt a little awkward. So I kissed them both, and we took a picture. It was the first picture of us since the one we took breaking camp at Lake Mead the morning of my accident.

I felt guilty about how those three seconds on the top of that wall radically changed my children's lives. They didn't choose to ride a motorcycle that day, and now I'd stacked the deck against them. How much harder had I made their teenage years? Instead of the typical supporting dad, they saw a guy reduced to a head on top of a functionless body.

I shudder to think what they must have thought while I was saying good-bye to them from the ditch and how this visit had scared them. All I had to offer them now was my love, support, and guidance. I'm proud of how they have survived and thrived through all these difficult times. I treasure them more than I can express with words.

# CHAPTER 35

# Don't Forget the Hands

While I could rest my arms around my kids' shoulders, I still couldn't flatten my hands out when my arms were extended, which was important to functionally using my hands and arms.

While most of our focus had been on walking, it was only half of my therapy. The other half was occupational therapy, which included working on relearning everyday tasks that are primarily performed with your arms, hands, and upper body. Occupational therapy was just as frustrating and every bit as exhausting as physical therapy.

The same heaviness and awkwardness that plagued my legs and feet also involved my hands and arms. I remember the first time I tried to put my hand on my face. My arm could not lift my hand all the way up, so they assisted my hand and rested it on my face. Because my hand was numb and I could hardly feel my arm, it felt like someone else's hand was on my face. It was the weirdest feeling. Logically, you know it's your hand on your face, but it doesn't feel like you.

There are different exercises in occupational therapy. One was exceptionally challenging for me. It involved picking up a metal ring off the table and putting it over a peg. Sounds simple enough, but not for me.

You have to be able to push your thumb against one end of the ring while your index finger gets the fingernail under the other side of the ring. Next, you have to pull up so you can get a second finger under the ring to grasp it.

If you get that far, it's time to engage your arm. Still gripping the ring with my gorilla hands, the shoulder had to lift up and maneuver the ring toward the peg. Once the ring is poised above the peg, you have to slowly lower it while keeping it horizontal. Even the slightest angle will keep it from fitting over the peg. When everything is finally lined up, you have a fraction of a second to let go. If something snags when you release, everything will be for naught. The ring will clang off to the side, and you have to start all over again.

It was grueling work for me. I didn't have fine motor control over my arm and hand muscles. My shoulder would get tired while I tried to line up the ring. The longer it took, the more tired I got. And the more tired I got, the harder it was to line up the ring to the peg. Often I had to drop my arm in fatigue before having a chance to release the ring.

The whole time, I was concentrating as though I was diffusing a bomb. When I was fortunate enough to be holding the ring over the peg, I had to contain my excitement. I was so close, but the possibility of success was so fleeting. When the ring slipped off, I was defeated. I'd let out a sigh as the therapist put the ring flat on the table again, and I'd start all over again.

It could take me 15 minutes before I felt the satisfaction of success. I'd smile broadly, resting my arm and relaxing my concentration. But my therapist didn't let me bask in my accomplishment. The ring came off the peg and she placed it back on the table.

The torture wasn't all about rings and pegs. Sometimes the occupational therapist devised other challenges for me. For instance, one morning they brought a nice plate of French toast into my room. I could smell it before I could even see what they were holding. Off came the plate cover, and there they were, the pieces of delectable toast waiting to melt on my tongue.

The catch? They told me I'd have to eat without assistance. In other words, if I wanted the toast in my mouth, I'd have to get it there by myself. It was terrible. I could see the tasty food inches from my face, but I couldn't get it. The smell made me salivate, and my body didn't understand why the wonderful sweetness was so far out of reach.

While I had been practicing with the ring and the peg, using a fork was a whole other matter. They have an apparatus that has a Velcro strap across the palm of your hand. There is a little holder on top for a utensil. They put a fork in that little pocket. The trick was learning how to rotate my wrist, stab the fork toward the pieces of bread, then hope to snag a piece well enough to keep the food on the fork.

Once the bread was properly impaled, I had to get it to my mouth, which was a whole other matter. My shoulder refused to follow a straight line from the plate to my mouth. I'd hold my mouth open as wide as possible as my hand wavered back and forth, trying to line up with my mouth. Then I had to bend my elbow at the correct angle to keep the food on the fork. When everything looked aligned, I rush the food toward my gaping mouth. When I got close, I'd bite at the food like I was a frog trying to catch a fly. Sometimes the fork would hit my chin instead of my mouth, dislodging the bite. The food was close enough to smell before it dropped to my chest.

Fortunately, I didn't have a shirt on because most of the food would fall off the fork and end up on my chest. I was left staring at the morsel, knowing I'd never have the opportunity to eat that one.

As more pieces landed on my chest, I began to despair that I would never get to taste the French toast. Worse, with fewer pieces on my plate, it became more and more difficult to stab one.

Throughout the process, the occupational therapist gave me instructions. Of course, I already knew what to do. I'd been feeding myself most of my life. But now I couldn't get my body to do what I wanted it to do.

Finally, a piece made it into my mouth. It was no longer warm, and now it was soggy, but that chunk of bread was tastier than anything I'd eaten before. I held it on my tongue, allowing it to dissolve.

Over time, I became more adept at getting food across the chasm between the plate and my mouth. Some foods were easier, like melons. I could stab them and they'd stay on the fork nicely. But burritos were another story.

Eventually, I got good enough at eating that they allowed me to take my meals in the lunch room. Being a sociable person, I like to interact with people when I eat. So I was excited that first day they wheeled me into the dinning room.

There were 30 or 40 others were already there. The therapist chose a table with only a few people at it. She sat down next to me to help.

I was so excited to be sitting up and eating like a real person that first day. I was concentrating on the process of getting food to my mouth, so I didn't interact with the other people at my table much more than greeting them. But over the next few days, I became more sociable. Usually, the people at the table would become uncomfortable watching me struggle. It would take about two minutes to get the food on a fork and lined up to my mouth. Then I'd have about a 40 percent success rate. The rest of the food would make a mess around me.

I would get so frustrated, even angry, but I held back because of the people eating at the table with me. If I didn't know the person, I'd break the ice with an old prison joke, asking, "What are you in here for?"

Everyone was curious about my situation, especially since I was one of the younger people at the hospital. Instead of letting them worry about how to ask about my injury, I would address the elephant in the room and offer, "I broke my neck on a motorcycle."

People reacted in different ways. Some didn't want to talk, which felt awkward, especially since eating was such a chore. And my occupational therapist didn't help matters because she didn't have a sense of humor. Worse, my charms didn't work on her, so I'd have to struggle in silence, aware that others were surreptitiously watching me.

Having played sports through high school, I understood there are coaches you respect but don't like. My occupational therapist was such a coach. She was good at what she did, and she pushed me to get better. I was thankful for that. But I also wanted my meals to be more enjoyable and social.

I didn't realize it at the time, but learning to use my hands would prove to be more useful than learning to walk. I regret that I never set "audacious" goals for using my hands. I never announced, "Today, I'm going to brush my teeth." While I would be walking across the threshold of my restaurant in the matter of months, it would take over a year to learn to brush my own teeth. And since my smile is the one thing I have going for me, learning to keep it clean and healthy is, ultimately, more important than walking across a threshold.

# CHAPTER 36

# Doctor Visit

For all those weeks of physical therapy and occupational therapy, with all the healing I was experiencing, I still did not know the exact nature of my injury, nor what had been done for me in surgery. In the haze of ICU, all I had learned was that there were no bones sticking into my spine, and that they were officially ruling my injury a spinal contusion.

What confused me was how my friend, Scott, could have a C1 break, drive himself to the hospital, and have no paralysis. And here I lay, struggling to move my limbs, and all I had was a concussed spine.

In my ninth week, I had an appointment with my surgeon. This was going to be my first time leaving Desert Canyon since I'd first come through their doors. I was excited to see Las Vegas and the outside world, even if it was while being strapped into a chair and having my head locked into place with my brace, stuck in the back of van. At least I'd be seeing my city and witnessing a world that most people took for granted.

They prepped me the morning of the appointment. Not only did they need to prepare me for the drive, but also for the longest time I'd been away from my bed. They told me it was important to stay cool and hydrated, so Megan packed a couple bottles of water for the drive. They gave me a bunch of other instructions, some I already knew, others were warnings in case different things happened.

I didn't do therapy that morning because they wanted me rested for the trip and the examination. So I was waiting, fully dressed and staring at the ceiling when the staff announced that the transportation van had arrived. They moved me to my Cadillac chair and took me down the hall and out the doors that acted as a gate to the outside world. I looked around quickly, knowing that my view would soon be restricted when they put me into the van.

Now, you'd assume these medical transportation drivers are medical professionals and that they understand the needs of the injured. But in reality, they have no medical training. They are just drivers with a certain amount of experience driving that particular van.

Putting me in the back was like securing a piece of cargo. Straps were secured to the floor with hooks on them, one for each corner of my wheelchair. Once those were cinched down, they put a shoulder belt across my chest and lap.

I watched the driver wipe sweat from his brow as he worked. It was a typical July day in Las Vegas with temperatures reaching into the triple digits.

Finally, I was locked down and the doors could be closed. Megan climbed into the passenger seat in front of me, ready for the ride.

A few minutes into the journey, the driver had to slam on the brakes because the light turned red sooner than expected. Because I didn't have a lot of control of my torso, I slid down with the forward motion of the van. I couldn't do anything as I began sliding underneath the shoulder restraint toward the floor. I cried out. " Stop! Stop! Stop! HELP!"

Megan jumped out of her seat and climbed over to me, trying to keep me from totally falling out of my chair. She started yelling at the driver, "Oh my God. I can't get him back in. I can't hold him. He's falling!"

The driver found a place to pull over and help Megan. He undid the restraints, counted to three, and hoisted me back into my chair. My heart was pounding. I had been in grave danger, and there was nothing I could do but watch my body slip out of the restraints. I could do nothing to protect myself as I slid toward the floor. I was like a rag doll falling. And who knows what would have happened had I fallen all the way out. Would I be injured? Could the two of them have gotten me back into the chair?

What was even more scary was watching Megan struggling with my size and weight. I could do nothing to help her. It underlined how dicey the entire situation was for us.

As we resumed the trip, the driver was more careful with the brakes. It was quiet and tense in the van. I know the thoughts that were going through Megan's head and mine; I can imagine what the driver was thinking, worrying about a report of the incident and what that would mean for his job. Each of us was relieved when we turned into the office complex where my surgeon was.

To get me out of the van, we had to reverse the process of getting me in. The driver undid the straps holding my chair. He then opened the side doors, and a blow-dryer like heat blasted me in the face. The hydraulic platform raised up to the level of the floor, nearly four feet off the ground. As he pushed me onto the platform, I realized that I was now at the same distance above the ground as I was when my motorcycle had been on that wall.

The driver locked the wheels of my chair and jumped down to lower the platform, leaving me up there by myself. It dawned on me that this was the first time I had been this far above the ground since the accident. And here I was, poised in another type of wheeled vehicle, at the exact vantage point I was that day, staring down at the pavement, alone, and now helpless. If I pitched forward, there was nothing I could do. I relived watching my front tire slip over the edge, propelling me forward.

I suddenly had an intense memory of my head hitting the concrete. It was so powerful, I had to close my eyes and grit my teeth. I could hear that sound again, and all the pain and fear of lying in the ditch, waiting for help to arrive.

The jolt of the ramp as it began to lower me made it worse. I didn't open my eyes until I felt the platform touch the ground. It was a visceral relief when my body sensed that the ramp was indeed resting on solid earth.

Once I was off the ramp and free of the van, the driver's responsibilities were over for the time being. It was up to Megan to get me to the doctor's office. Gallantly, she began pushing me. We faced a ramp leading from the parking level to the front doors. To this point, she had only pushed me along level hallways; now she had to push all this weight uphill, all the way to the entrance. I couldn't see her struggling behind me, but I could imagine her braced with her body forward, head down, and legs straining to get this big man and his heavy chair all the way up.

I do know she was breathing hard when we paused at the top to push the button for the automatic doors. While we waited, she had the posture of a sprinter resting between meets.

Once inside, things didn't get easier for her. Sure, we were on the level, but now we had carpet. In the hospital, we had highly polished floors, but carpet was a whole other issue. I could hear Megan breathing hard behind me. When she'd tire and need to reposition her grip, our progress would stop all together. Then she'd have to get what little momentum she could all over again.

It was humbling for me to hear her straining while I could do nothing to help out. Before the accident, my size allowed me to be able to take care of myself and to help other people. Now I was completely dependent on this slight lady. It's not my nature to have other people help me. I'd been an independent person, taking care of whatever needs or wants I had. Now, I couldn't be chivalrous enough to help Megan. Worse, I was the cause of all her struggles.

Finally, we were at the doctor's office. We were late, but only by minutes. I thought we'd have a special pass. I expected them to treat me like a VIP approaching the velvet rope. "Hello, Mr. Frost. Right this way." After all, I was paralyzed and we'd worked hard to get there.

But we had no such luck. We were just like everyone else in the waiting room. We had to fill out all the forms and go through the formalities of doctors' offices. Then we had to wait just like everyone else.

When you count the drive and now the waiting room, I had been upright for several hours. This was putting stress on my body, which wanted to be lying down. And yet, we were left watching the time pass. The difference for me was I might soon pass out. The others in the roomy were simply inconvenienced by the wait.

When the surgeon did finally see us, I had the first opportunity to ask about my injury and what he'd done during surgery. He told me he had removed the disk between C3 and C4. When my head snapped backward, the crushed disk pushed forward into the back of my spine, robbing it of valuable oxygen. So it had to be removed to take the pressure off the spinal cord. They put bone putty where the disk was, and small plastic stints on each side of the spine. Next, they put in brackets and screws to fuse the C3 and C4 vertebras into place.

Unbeknownst to me, they had taken X-rays after my surgery. When my surgeon mentioned the X-rays, I was eager to see them. He put them up on the back-light viewer. It took my breath away. The screws were huge.

He explained the nature of my injury and how spine injuries are like snowflakes, everyone of them is different. Some people can break vertebrae, but as long as their spine is not contused or there was nothing puncturing or putting pressure on the spine, no paralysis would take place. In my instance, my spine had been compressed and bent straight backward. This had crushed the disk, pushing it forward. Those three elements are what caused the paralysis.

I asked the doctor what he thought my prognosis would be. Everyone always asked me what "they" say about my future. The closest thing to "they" was my surgeon. I figured whatever he said would be what I'd tell people.

He asked me if I had been able to move anything. I raised my hands and wiggled my toes for him. He lit up, slapped me on the thigh, and said, "Ah, you're going to be fine." Then he left the room.

I stared at the now closed door. I wasn't sure what "fine" meant, but I took it as a good sign.

With that, it was time to get me back to Desert Canyon. It was 5:30, more than three and a half hours since we left Desert Canyon. And it was 112 degrees outside.

As we merged onto the freeway, traffic slowed to a crawl. Going that slowly, in that much heat, with so much internal space to keep cool in the van, the air conditioner couldn't keep up.

As it got warmer in the van, my body didn't have a mechanism to deal with the heat. Messages about body temperature weren't reaching my brain. There was no signal telling my brain to start sweating to keep my core temperature down.

Looking back to check on me, Megan could see that something was wrong. All we had to help keep me cool was a couple bottles of water. She threw the water on me and fanned me, trying to cool me down.

We had been warned about the heat, but I guess everyone assumed the van would be air conditioned enough to keep me safe. Instead, I was cooking in the van, and my body had no way to deal with it. Megan did her best to cool me down, but we only had two bottles of water and traffic wasn't moving.

I was in bad shape by the time we reached Desert Canyon. Once again, the driver, not thinking about my injury, unloaded me facing directly into the sun. The whole process of unloading took about five minutes and now I didn't have the advantage of what little cooling the van's air conditioner gave. My eye's rolled into the back of my head, and I lost consciousness.

The head nurse came out, took one look at me, and rushed me inside.

The driver yelled, "Hey, you have to do the paperwork first." She ignored him.

My blood pressure was 60 over 40. They elevated my feet and packed me in ice. They worked on me for a good 15 minutes before my blood pressure returned and I regained consciousness.

Everyone at Desert Canyon was emphatic that from now on, where ever I go, I need to take ice, water, and rags. Just a few moments of heat, and I could die of heat stroke. We'd had another close call, and the lesson was learned.

# CHAPTER 37

# Time to Leave

It was now nearly three months after my accident, and my progress began to level off. The major gains were no longer coming, though I continued to make small, incremental progress. I was able to stand in my platform walker a little longer, step a little more smoothly even though I had no balance. I could reliably grip a utensil, but getting it to my mouth was still a 50/50 proposition. And I could still not bathe myself, brush my teeth, sit up, rollover, get out of bed, dress, or go to the bathroom by myself. Even though I could move, which I was thankful for, I was still 100 percent reliant on those around me.

With my continued limitations, I had a certain comfort knowing that there was a staff of nurses and therapists around to assist my family and me. Things began to fall into a routine. They'd get me up, I'd work hard in therapy, then fall into a power coma. When I woke up, it was time to struggle through occupational therapy. When I was done with that, it was time for dinner. And then I'd spend the evening with Megan.

For all the comfort of the routine, in the back of my mind I knew there would come a time to leave. Until that time came, though, I didn't want to worry about what would happen next.

But then the hospital officials started saying things like, "It looks like you are leveling out," or "When you get ready to go..."

Whenever the caseworker showed up, we knew she wasn't dropping by to see how I was doing. Something was up. Her job was to make sure the hospital gets paid, not to advocate for my continued care.

Back when my 30 days were about up, and the insurance company said they'd keep paying my bill, she was incredulous, almost indignant. She was like, "What makes you so special?" With an attitude like that, we had a tense relationship over the months I was in the hospital.

Then one day, she called Megan and me into her office and said, "We need to go over your discharge papers."

When I heard that, I said, "Are you kidding me?"

There has to be a better way of letting people know they are about to get kicked out of a facility. Don't tell me on a Wednesday that I have to be out by Friday. Give me a week, at least. People need time to prepare both emotionally and practically.

I discovered that, on a weekly basis, the therapists had to score me on a scale known as an FIM Score. This was then reported to the insurance company, and the insurance company would grant me one more week of therapy according to my FIM scores.

My FIM scores, apparently, had plateaued. I wish I would have known I was being measured like this and what specific goals I was shooting for in my therapy. Had I known the criteria, I would have been sure to push for the score I needed for each specific measurement. Instead, I had stubbornly pushed the envelope on walking. It turns out, walking wasn't the most important thing they were measuring.

The case worker pushed papers in front of me. "Sign these."

Of course, I couldn't sign my name. I could barely keep a pen between my fingers. She sat back while Megan put the pen in hand like a knife, and I struggled to make a squiggly "X." Then I angrily dropped the pen. Obviously, I wasn't ready to take care of myself.

"What's next?" I asked.

She said, "You have until the end of the week."

I shook my head in disgust.

Megan wheeled me out of her office and we went back to the room that had been home for the last three months. We looked around and then at each other. We were scared to leave the space. We'd gone through so much there, both painful and beautiful. We had discovered what was really important in life: My faith, my family, my friends, my business, and the opportunity to live a life with a new perspective. And now we were going to leave the safety of this room.

I had to break the news to my parents. This was going to be burdensome to everyone around me. The major concern was whether my family would be able to care for me adequately and safely. Megan and my father had helped the nurses, but I couldn't only rely on them. Megan was still working, and my dad couldn't be my sole caregiver when she was out.

My mom, for all her willingness to help, is too small of a person to pull me up or hold me when I am standing. It takes a lot of leverage and muscle to get this lump of flesh to where it needs to go.

I called my parents and broke the news. It was overwhelming, I'm sure, but we got down to business. We made a plan right there on the phone. Megan and I looked around my hospital room, listing all the things we would need: hospital bed, a shower/bathroom chair, transportation, at-home therapy, and everything that went with taking care of a quadriplegic. It was a long list.

With 48 hours to go before my discharge, we had a dry run where everyone gathered around and took turns using the right biomechanics to sit me up in bed and help me stand up. They learned how to put me into bed safely, how to transfer me from the bed to the wheelchair, and vice versa. Even the kids had to learn how to brace me and pull me out of the chair. Everyone learned how to strap the gait belt around my torso, how to maneuver my limbs, what to check for in my care, the different medications I was taking, and on and on. We also went through different scenarios like, "If he's up in his walker and starts to fall, what do you do?"

It was haphazard training and a stop-gap that made the hospital officials feel better about sending me out the door. But everyone knew in their hearts that my family could not provide even close to the level of care the hospital staff had been giving me.

In the midst of this, Megan had to make a choice. She had graduated from the University of Nevada, Las Vegas, and had gotten her dream job with Limited Brands. She'd been working with them for a little over a year. But with all that was going to be required to care for me, we knew my father couldn't be my sole caregiver. At 25, Megan had to choose between her career and being a caregiver. It made me sick to put such a huge decision on her.

Megan ended up taking a paid leave of absence. She was allowed up to 90 days. We decided to give it those 90 days to see what would happen with me, and then make a final decision.

Our last night in the hospital was peaceful. Megan had packed everything up. She took down the posters and cards. And we spent the evening looking at all the pictures and videos we'd taken since the accident on her digital camera. We reflected on how close we had become and the incredible miracles that had happened.

I asked her, "Can you imagine if this hadn't happened? Where we would be?"

She looked at me, "I wouldn't be here."

"I'm glad you are. Thank you for sticking with me."

It was another way that God's plan had manifested itself, the fact that Megan and I were still together.

"So would you like to make this living arrangement permanent?" I asked.

She nodded.

I looked at her, those beautiful green eyes. "The day I can stand through our wedding ceremony is the day I'll marry you."

Once again, I had set an audacious goal. And this one I swore I would keep.

The next morning was hectic. There were so many last minute considerations. Things would pop up that we hadn't thought of. And then there was the paper work. Underlying all of the activity was the stress of not knowing how I would live outside of the hospital. There were so many unknowns.

I was exhilarated and scared at the same time. We were leaving the safe haven of the hospital and nurses, and moving on with the rest of our lives. Talk about having to put your trust in God. I didn't know what life outside the hospital would look like, how my family would be able to deal with my physical inabilities, or how we would cover our living expenses, not to mention the medical costs.

As we rushed to get things ready for my departure, I reminded Megan that my first audacious goal was that I would walk out of the hospital. I couldn't walk on my own, but I could use my walker.

Word spread among the staff that I would be leaving that day. One by one, the people I had been working so hard with, those who had taken such good care of me, stopped by. It was emotional; there were tears and laughter.

One of the side effects of my mediation was dry mouth, so months earlier, I had Megan buy Lemonheads candy. They were sour, which kept my mouth from feeling dry, especially during therapy. It became protocol to have a box of the candies at rehab.

So the staff went online and found a Lemonheads T-shirt for me. They presented it to me that morning, so I could wear it out the door. I couldn't think of a better send-off gift. I was proud to wear that shirt on my day of transition from hospital to home.

And then it was time. The good-byes were over and I had to leave the confines of the hospital behind. I was being wheeled out of a room that would soon be someone else's, probably in a matter of hours after I was gone. That person wouldn't know about me, nor my experiences at Desert Canyon.

They wheeled me to the threshold, braced me up, and slung me in the platform walker. I paused for dramatic effect, and then walked out the door of the hospital on my own two feet.

An audacious goal and a lot of effort had been rewarded with a miracle. This paralyzed man was walking on his own two feet out of the hospital when everyone else thought he would only leave on a stretcher. I was exceedingly grateful for what God had given me.

As I stepped on the ground outside the hospital door, I said, "Get ready, world. It's Scott Frost, Version 2.0."

# CHAPTER 38

# Moving Back Home

It was nerve-wracking setting up a new life. My house was only 1300 square feet with three bedrooms and two bathrooms upstairs and a half bath downstairs. Besides me and Megan, we had two kids, and now my parents staying in the house. And let's not forget the family dog, Mickey, our beloved Jack Russel terrier. He was a dead-ringer for the dog on the television show *Frasier*.

The house wasn't designed for a paralyzed person. The bedrooms and bathrooms were upstairs, and I couldn't climb the stairs. And even if I could, it would be difficult getting my hospital bed up there. So, we put my hospital bed in the living room. Megan slept on the couch next to me. Taylor kept her old room, and my mother took over the master bedroom. Originally, Christian was in his room with my dad, but my dad snores so badly, even Christian couldn't handle it. So he moved downstairs and slept on an air mattress near Megan and me.

It's hard to believe how cramped we were, not just because of the small amount of living space for so many people, but also because of all the space I needed. The hospital bed was gigantic and took up most of the living room. Add to that all the other medical equipment and the house was cluttered, to say the least.

The other issue was there was only a half-bath on the main floor. Since it took two people to get me on the toilet, we all couldn't fit in the small room. So we had to set up a commode in the living room. It was a big plastic bench with a hole in the middle and a handle on each side. There was a bucket that slid underneath the hole under the bench. I chuckled to myself when I thought of the old saying, "You shouldn't crap where you sleep," but here I was literally doing just that. I had no choice.

The good news is that my mom had cleaned the house before I came home. The last time I had been in the house, it was a disaster area. My surroundings matched my state of mind before the accident. I had been miserable without Megan. I hadn't cleaned, filed the mail, or done the laundry in weeks. Coming home that day, it was great seeing the house looking nice. I felt comfortable having my parents and children living there.

Before the accident, my children and I called the house our "healing house." As a family, we had recovered from the divorce in that home. We'd gotten family counseling there. It also was the house where I started my company. There were a lot of good memories under that roof.

This house was going to continue being a healing house, only now it was going to be about physical healing. It wasn't going to be easy. There were a lot of challenges ahead that involved my physical incapacities and needs. Transferring me from bed to chair or from bed to commode was tough. Megan, my dad, or one of the kids had to be present at all times.

When you're paralyzed, all privacy and modesty go out the window. Often, the urge to go number two came unexpectedly. Someone had to be nearby to maneuver me out of bed on onto my commode. It proved to be a hit or miss proposition.

When I left the house that Sunday of the accident, I hadn't anticipated that I'd be returning in a wheelchair. Furniture had to be removed. Paths through the house had to be created. And the rest of the family still had to be able to live in the house.

Since there wasn't a way to get me upstairs to the tubs, and there weren't any facilities on the main floor, we had to think outside the box, literally.

I looked around the downstairs, and then out the back door. We didn't have space inside, so maybe outside? We could wheel me out there, and use a hose or something. But we had a typical Vegas lot with two-story houses all around, looking into each others' backyards. The neighbors could see me naked and helpless being hosed down.

If not the back, how about the front? My front porch had a type of portico covering the front door. There was an archway and a few feet to the actual door. Why not turn it into a shower?

We hung a shower curtain from the archway. Since it was a small space designed to simply give shade to those waiting at the front door, Megan and my dad had to wheel me out onto the front porch fully dressed. Then they put up the shower curtain. Then they'd wheel me behind the curtain, all three of us were crammed between the front door and the shower curtain. Next, they'd stand me up to undress me. Sit me down, now naked, on my commode because it was the only "chair" that could get wet.

Finally, we were ready for the hose. We ran it from the kitchen sink, so at least it was warm. I was spending a lot of time naked, outdoors, some of it wet. Without warm water, it would be difficult to clean me before my body temperature dropped. Plus, it was difficult to clean me without Megan getting wet as well. Since, at that point, I couldn't even touch the top of my head, Megan had to do all the washing. It was a mess with the hose running, soap everywhere. It was sort of like washing a car on your front porch.

To dry me off, Megan and my father would stand me up. I would hold onto the platform walker as they toweled me down while making sure I stayed upright and didn't fall. Once I was dry, they would put me naked back into my wheelchair, wheel me inside, and dress me.

Then they'd go back outside, take down the shower curtain, unhook the hose from the sink, and clean up the front porch. It was quite a process.

I often wondered what my neighbors would think if they saw this routine. My mom worried they'd report us to the home owners association. I'm pretty sure showering on the front porch was not allowed.

I reasoned with her that our neighbors, if anything, would feel sorry for us. They wouldn't report us. Besides, we didn't have an alternative.

When I was at the inpatient facility, everything was at my fingertips. Nurses were there at my beck and call. Anything I needed would be provided. And everything in my surroundings was there to accommodate my injuries.

I can't imagine what it was like from my family's perspective once we were all in the house. Every once in a while, I put myself in my father's shoes. He was in his 70s. After 20 years in the army and a second career as a college administrator, he'd had a life of hard work. Before my accident, he was enjoying retirement. And now he was responsible for lifting his son onto the toilet and cleaning him afterward. I don't know how he did it. He's a strong man.

And my mom, decades had gone by since she'd last had to care for her children. She too had worked hard her entire life, including 35 years as a teacher. Like my father, she had been enjoying retirement. Now, she was feeding me like I was an infant, and cleaning and cooking for three generations in my little house.

Megan was keeping the whole family together. And while she had lived with my children and me for two years before the accident, she was now thrust into a situation she hadn't prepared for. At 25 years old, she was managing my care and making sure everyone was as comfortable as possible.

And the kids. No child should have to care for their parent the way my children have. Just the fact that I was reduced to using the commode in the living room, feet away from Christian's bed, says a lot about the situation they were in. They should have had the opportunity to be typical, self-centered teenagers. Instead, they had to care for their father and modify their lives to accommodate his physical condition.

Everyone likes to praise me for how far I've come and the struggles I've had, but I say, "Look at the people around me. They are the ones who are brave and inspiring. I would have to be a total jackass if I didn't try hard after all they've done for me."

Despite all the adversity, everyone in my family fell into their roles when we returned home. We learned to accept each others' emotional highs and lows, as well as the inevitable physical exhaustion that came with our situation. I prayed hard every night that this family would continue to pull together and be able to withstand the hardships we all faced.

I'm proud of my family. No one complained, and everyone pulled together to do their part. My family is a true blessing, a blessing I would not have appreciated had I not been so dependent on them.

# CHAPTER 39

# At-Home Therapy

Now that I was out of the hospital, my biggest fear was that I would lose the momentum I had going with my physical recovery. I was used to having therapy everyday. It was a luxury having a staff dedicated to my physical wellbeing and development at Desert Canyon. Now, we were on our own.

I began working with a physical therapist and an occupational therapist in my home several days a week. I didn't have all the equipment I'd had in the hospital, and the sessions weren't as intense. It was up to me to push and continue to make progress.

For instance, I didn't have parallel bars in our little house, nor weights, nor a 300 ft. hallway to walk down. Instead of being strapped into a specialized machine, my physical therapy consisted of learning how to push off the arms of my chair and stand up without having to be pulled up. We worked on leg strength and arm strength in the confines of my house. All we could do was multiple reps of exercises. I'd sit up, stand up, sit down, stand up, and take a step forward, take one backward, take one forward again. I'd also do laps in our short hallway. It was difficult since I had to make 180 degree turns for each lap.

My occupational therapist had me working with exercise bands and arm weights. She also had me doing various exercises with my hands to improve my dexterity. My shoulders were still "frozen" from the accident. My range of motion limited my ability to reach for things. She would stretch my shoulders to the point of intense pain. She admonished my family for not stretching me more on the days she wasn't there. Of course, with the pain this stretching was causing me, only the most hardened person could do what she was expecting. She was tough.

One day, I was complaining to the physical therapist about the occupational therapist. I told him she didn't understand the situation.

"You don't like her?" he asked.

"I don't like her accusing me of not trying hard enough." I said. "Compared to you, she's not very nice."

He said, "I'll have to tell her that tonight."

Confused, I asked, "Huh?

He repeated, "I'll have to tell my wife tonight.

"You two are married?"

"Yeah," he smiled, knowing he had pushed me into complaining about her.

It turns out they were a tag-team at-home physical and occupational therapist service who happened to be married.

I chuckled. What a way to find out.

My body was still healing, so even if the sessions weren't as intense in my house, I was still struggling and pushing myself to improve. And this took energy. After my therapy sessions, I'd still fall into a power coma. One minute I would be talking to someone, and the next minute I'd be out cold, snoozing away.

Despite all of this activity and the resultant power comas, I had work to do. We were in the design and construction phases of the restaurant and nightclub. A couple times a week, I'd go into the office. Either Meg or my dad would drive me over in my van, and I'd try to stay awake as long as possible, usually sleeping on the way back to the house after meetings with my staff and vendors, and dealing with all the tasks that go into opening a restaurant and a night club at the same time.

We had a new normal. In the old days, I could sleep in as late as possible, rush everyone out the door and head to work. Now it took hours to prepare for anything, even the smallest appointment or phone call. Loading me into and out of the van took a long time. When we finally got to work, I had a limited amount of time before my body began shutting down. Just when I felt like I was getting things done, we'd have to head home to rest and recover from the day. It was frustrating to fight against my limitations. There was so much I had to do, but when my body was done, it was done. I had to learn to accept it.

There is a lot I've learned from being a good patient and going through therapy that made me a better boss. I got really good at giving clear directions, describing my thoughts and ideas, building teams, motivating people, and not micromanaging the process. I learned quickly that I had to focus on outcomes and end-goals. This was all a completely different approach than I had before the accident. Back then, I didn't delegate, I didn't support my team, and I managed by command. But when I had physical limitations, I learned to be a true leader. I had to adjust my entire thought process and become more strategically oriented and leave the tactical implementations to my team.

This was yet another paradoxical result of my accident: had it not happened, I would not be the effective businessman and leader that I am today. Imagine if I could have learned these business lessons without breaking my neck. I would have had the skills of leadership with the physical capabilities I had before the accident.

There was a lot of work and struggle in those first weeks and months at home. It seemed like every waking moment was filled with something, whether therapy, work, or preparing me to go somewhere or bringing me home and settling me back into bed. For a man who spent most of his time either in bed or in a chair, I sure was busy.

# CHAPTER 40

# Generosity

There is a financial reality with health care. It didn't take long before the bills started arriving. We ignored the early threats of payment, waiting for the insurance company to sort out all the claims. But there came a time when we had to face the bills that would not be covered. The helicopter flight that eventually took me to the hospital after the accident cost $19,000. My ICU bill for just my stay was $185,000. The surgery was a separate bill that was close to $50,000. And there were other bills for things like the anesthesiologist, equipment charges, and so on. We were left wondering how we could ever pay for everything.

Yes, we had insurance, but there was still plenty that was not covered. And we had no idea how we would cover even 10% of the total bill.

My friends understood that we would be in financial strain, and they wanted to help. So the Committee set up a website to take donations to make it easier for people to give money to help with my health-care bills. It was amazing to see how people I barely knew, even complete strangers, made donations over the Internet. Transactions were coming from all over the place, even internationally. I was humbled and honored.

The first guy to donate at our website sent me $100. I grew up with him, and he was the last person I thought would help. He had been a bully in high school, a loud mouth, and I didn't like him. It turned out he was now a recovering alcoholic and had gained a new perspective on life. He wanted to express his regret for transgressions that happened decades in the past. It felt weird to accept his generous gift, but in my situation, I was thankful for the help and support.

That day, a successful friend of mine stopped by. He asked me how things were going. I told him how excited I was that the childhood acquaintance had just donated $100.

Jeff asked, "$100? Is that your biggest donation?"

I said, "Yes, so far."

"Let me get on the phone," he responded.

Three days later, he handed me a check for $15,000.

Jeff had rounded up some of my friends in my entrepreneur group, and they had pooled their resources to come up with the $15,000. I was so happy. Here I was, wondering how I was going to pay for everything, and once again, God put somebody in front of me who I didn't expect to help. Sometimes the shortest prayer you can say is "Help."

With the website set up and donations coming in, the Committee focused their attentions on a fundraiser for me. They approached a friend of mine, Kerry Simon, who was a popular chef in Las Vegas. He graciously donated his banquet space and the pool area around his restaurant at the Palms Resort Casino. That wasn't all he did; he agreed to have a no-host bar and put out free food for my guests.

The Committee then approached people I knew and had done business with to ask for donations to the silent auction.

These people graciously donated items and services that cost them real dollars and required them to donate hours of service. Other friends and family volunteered to help out with the fundraiser.

I was humbled that this huge event was being put on in my honor, and all I had to do was show up.

Which wasn't as easy as it may sound. At that point, I was taking three to four naps a day. I couldn't stay awake more than a few hours at a time. I knew I'd have to put out a lot of energy to talk with the people who were there to support me.

My doctor didn't condone the event. I had just gotten out of the neck brace, and he was worried I'd re-injure myself. He also wasn't keen on me being outside and talking for that long. But with so many people giving to me, I was determined to give back to them.

When we arrived at Kerry's restaurant, more than a hundred people were gathered around the pool and throughout the restaurant. The DJ was pumping music, and people were meeting each other and catching up.

I was amazed, honored, and humbled by all the people who showed up. People were there from different circles of my life. I even had a friend from high school, who I hadn't seen in years, surprise me. He happened to be in town for a convention, and had heard about the fundraiser from a mutual friend. It was amazing to see him meeting people from my different business circles and acquaintances. With him there, I had representation from pretty much every aspect of my life.

It was like attending your own funeral. I had the opportunity to have all my friends and family in one place, talking about how much I meant to them, and sharing stories about crazy things we'd done together. It had a profound affect on me. I could never have seen all of these people again, but here I was, lucky enough to not only see them, but hear exactly what I had meant to them, and see how happy they were to have me in their lives.

Relationships are something I will never take for granted again.

There were still so many people to talk with when Megan wheeled me outside where they had a microphone ready for me. I thanked everyone for coming out. Then I did my best to talk with everyone one-on-one. I couldn't talk fast enough or long enough. I was there for a solid two hours. I was fading at the end, but the love and affection everyone was showing me, buoyed me up. I couldn't believe the generosity people were showing me.

The suggested donation for the night was $100. I know of one person who gave $700, and I also know she couldn't afford that much. Another person donated $1,000. Plus there were those who donated items and services to a silent auction which sold out.

By the end of the night, we raised close to $17,000. I can't express my amazement at their generosity.

When is first in the hospital, I made a conscious decision not to ask why this was happening to me; instead, I focused on how was I going to make it work. After that decision, things began to unfold. I learned a valuable lesson: You have to give to get. If you give your best to others, they'll surprise you by how much they will give back. That night at Simon's Restaurant, I felt that I got back way more than I'd given over the years.

Of course, now that they had helped me, it was important that I not let them down. Many of those gathered gave more than they could afford. If they were going to make that kind of investment in me, I had better make sure their money went a long way toward my healing. The bar was raised with the outpouring of affection. I felt an obligation to stay upbeat, continue to run my business, hold my family together, and be the best man I could be.

# CHAPTER 41

# Hussong's Cantina

If you've never opened a business before, it's tough to imagine all the difficulties, obstacles, details, last-minute changes, and the unexpected issues that have to be addressed in the months and weeks before an opening. My team had opened night clubs before, and others had worked in restaurants, but we discovered opening a restaurant is a whole other matter.

Before the accident, the opportunity to open Hussong's Cantina in Las Vegas was a typical business opportunity for my company. Like any business, we were constantly looking to grow. Under normal circumstances, it would have been stressful and challenging to capitalize on this opportunity. But then my accident happened. Now opening the restaurant was an even more arduous undertaking. Plus, I had added the audacious goal of walking into the restaurant opening night to order the first margarita.

Every couple of days, Megan would load me into the van and take me down to the restaurant so I could check on the progress of construction. Walls were getting torn down, new ones put up, the kitchen equipment was being installed, and the bar was being built. Since we were staying true to the original Hussong's, the decor had to be just right. And there were a myriad of other details that had to be addressed.

We hired our executive chef, Noe. I worked with him to begin hiring kitchen staff well before we opened. My partners, MJ and Brian, also interviewed and hired the house staff. All of us were feeling our way along, unsure of exactly what we'd need and who we would need to have a successful opening.

At home, we intensified my therapy. When we were months away from the opening, we began to focus on walking without the use of the platform walker. My therapist had me experimenting with crutches, and even had me use a single four-prong cane. I was able to do this, but it was flat out not safe.

After discussing it with my therapist, we decided it would be best for the opening-night walk to use a hand-held assist. I would stand up and Megan would hold my left hand. I would slowly take steps and rely on her to keep my balance. This too was a dicey maneuver, but I felt more comfortable relying on Megan than trying to use the cane all by myself.

Once the bar was constructed, we measured the distance from the bar's closest corner to the front of the restaurant. We then added a few extra feet since I would be starting my walk in the mall at the Shops of Mandalay Bay. It was 28 feet.

That may not sound like a lot, but once we had it as a therapeutic goal, I discovered that it is a long way, especially with the difficulty I had getting my left leg forward. We also had to anticipate all the distractions of well-wishers, the noise of an celebration, and even the surge of adrenaline I would get.

Once I made the 28 feet the first time, we knew it wasn't enough. I practiced day after day, over and over again. This was a goal that would take a lot of work to prepare for and one I couldn't fail.

As opening day approached, it felt like we needed another month to get all the details ironed out. There were meetings after meetings, arguments over every detail, and so many moving parts. On top of all this, I was still rehabing. The added stress of work made my "power comas" more frequent. I knew they were part of my healing process, but it was so frustrating to get tired that often.

Suddenly it was opening day. There was no turning back, no request for an extra day or two, no chance to back away from my audacious goal.

About 200 friends and family were at the opening. And since we'd hyped the opening, and the angle that I would be walking across the threshold, up to the bar, and ordering the first margarita, the press was also there. Not just the local press, the *LA Times* had also written an article about my pending feat and the opening of the restaurant. Talk about pressure. "Me and my big mouth," I thought. Then I remembered who had given me the strength each time I had blurted out one of my audacious goals. I thought back to that night when I heard the message. This was my opportunity to inspire everyone in the crowd.

The original Hussong's Cantina was established in 1892 in Ensenada, Mexico. In 1941, bartender Don Carlos Orozco invented the margarita for a beautiful woman rumored to be Rita Hayworth. The reason I wanted to order the first margarita at the Las Vegas iteration of Hussong's was to acknowledge the heritage and to continue the legacy of the restaurant.

When the grand opening began, I sat outside greeting everyone as they arrived. It was great to see everyone, many of whom I hadn't seen since the accident. It was a mixture of "how are you?" and questions about the restaurant. Sitting there, I was nervous, anxious, and excited.

About an hour into the grand opening, it was finally time. MJ, our director of operations, got on the microphone and introduced me. "For the first time in a long time, Scott is going to walk with his girlfriend. He's going to come to the bar, and order the first margarita."

Silence blanketed the crowd. All eyes turned toward me in my wheelchair in the mall, facing toward the bar. The crowd parted to create a aisle that reminded me of the spirit tunnels my high school football teams used to run through on our way onto the field. I was flanked by a marriachi band complete with trumpets, guitars, and a chorus of singers.

That 28 feet that I'd walked so many times before in practice seemed like a quarter mile. In the distance, I could see the bartender waiting to make me that first drink. I couldn't help but smile because a drink at the end of the bar was always a great motivator for me. But it had never been this hard to get one.

I took a deep breath and pressed down with my arms and pushed up with my legs, slowly standing up. People began cheering and clapping. I grabbed Megan's hand. I looked her in the eye and smiled. I could tell she was concerned. At this point, I needed her emotional support more than her physical support.

From where I stood up, I had four feet to walk just to get to the threshold. Those first steps seemed to take forever. Right foot forward, transfer the weight, press down on Megan's hand, slide the left foot forward, anchor it, shift the weight, step the right forward, and repeat. Inch by slow, laborious inch.

I approached the threshold. I paused to make that first step. As soon as it landed, the mariachi band began playing. A trumpet blasted right in my face.

I stumbled slightly with the surprise of the horn blast. I stopped walking to steady myself, but I made it look like I meant to pause for dramatic effect. I smiled and gave everyone a thumbs up. Little did they know, I was genuinely afraid of falling. The guests cheered even louder. I fed off their goodwill and continued my journey.

My goal was in sight. Twelve feet, step, step. Five feet, step, step. Two feet. I'm almost there. I reached out my right hand to the bar to steady myself.

Finally, I was at the bar. They placed a bar stool behind me, and I sat down.

I motioned with my index finger to the bartender like I was ordering one drink. The crowd erupted. I'd made it, another audacious goal reached, and this one in front of my friends, family, and the media.

I looked at Megan. She looked into my eyes. All of a sudden, everything that had happened over the last eight months washed over me. She put her hand behind my head and pulled her forehead to mine. All the hard work, all the tears, all the pain, all the fear, all the doubt, all the worry, it all came flashing across my eyes. A huge weight lifted off me.

I started sobbing. I curled my head down into Megan and just let the tears flow. People were patting me on the back while I shook with sobs.

When I recovered my emotions, and my drink was in front of me, I lifted my head and smiled at the crowd. They put a long straw in the glass, I leaned forward and took the first sip in my new restaurant. Everyone cheered again.

Then they handed me the microphone. Over the noise of the crowd, I shouted, "This is what life is about, what you just saw. It's not about accumulating wealth, cars, houses; it's about moments like this, surrounded by friends and family. This is what it's all about."

It was quite a journey from a dusty motorcycle ride to that bar stool. I'd learned a lot about myself. I'd become a better person, and I still had a long ways to go, but at the moment, I knew I was going to be okay. I couldn't imagine the difficult times that lay ahead, but I knew I had the strength to handle them. I quietly thanked God for it all.

# CHAPTER 42

# The Biggest Miracle of All

Now that the restaurant was open, we were beginning a new chapter in our lives. I was no longer a patient. I would always be struggling with my body, but it was no longer the focal point of our existence.

We began to focus on being a family again. Christian and Taylor were still in high school. Once they were assured that I was going to be okay, they began treating me like a regular parent. Just as any teenagers would, they tested the boundaries of my patience. They also went through the typical struggles that teenagers in high school do.

Megan and I started to socialize again outside of the house, going to concerts and movies, going out to dinner with other people and visiting friends in their homes.

During the week, we had an office to go to and a business to run. And the prospect of growing the company kept me engaged and focused.

My parents did one of the most selfless things a parent could do; they helped me buy a new house that we could all live in. I no longer had to take porch showers and everyone had their own rooms. I realized that no matter how old you are, as long as you have kids, you never stop being a parent.

The last night in the hospital, I had promised Megan that when I was able to stand throughout our wedding ceremony, I would put a ring on her finger and marry her. It wasn't your typical proposal. I certainly couldn't have gotten down on a knee. It was more of a commitment to her and a declaration of an even more important audacious goal. We didn't tell anybody about our commitment, nor did I begin referring to her as my fiance.

We hadn't set a date, because the goal was dependent on my physical progress. But we did begin thinking about significant dates. In the 2000s, throngs of people were getting married on repeating dates like 08/08/08 and 09/09/09. The next significant date like this was 10/10/10. In conversations, we said, "Hey, we should get married on 10/10/10," almost in passing.

During all the excitement surrounding the opening of Hussong's, a reporter from the *Las Vegas Review Journal* wanted to do a story about Megan and me.

When the reporter was interviewing us, we let it slip that we were going to be getting married on 10/10/10. After that revelation, it felt weird to refer to Megan in the article as my girlfriend, so I called her my fiance for the first time.

Once we wrapped up the interview, the reporter let us know that the article would be published that Friday, just two days later. We thanked the reporter and looked forward to reading the article.

Late Thursday night, we realized that people were going to hear that we were engaged from the newspaper. They would be upset and hurt that we didn't tell them in person. More importantly, we knew Megan's dad was an early riser and an avid reader of the paper. If he read the article before we told him, he would be upset. It was now midnight.

We quickly got on the phone and called Megan's parents. We freaked them out because we were calling so late.

"What's wrong?" they asked. "Are you okay?"

We told them we were fine, and that we were actually calling with good news. We are getting married on 10/10/10.

Despite being upset for alarming them by calling in the middle of night, they wearily congratulated us. Then they told us to go to bed.

Now that we had set a date, I worked on strengthening my core and leg muscles so I'd be able to stand for a length of time. And of course I kept working on walking longer and longer distances with Megan holding my hand. The looming date added a sense of urgency.

At one point, as wedding plans began to get complicated, Megan wanted to elope. She was never one for big fairy-tale weddings, and she hates being the center of attention.

I objected, saying, "Hey, I'm a dad. I know that I'd be upset if my baby girl eloped. Your dad would kill me first, and then you, if we eloped."

Instead, we planned a small ceremony in the chapel of our church. It would be an intimate and poignant affair.

We were less than a month away from our wedding; I was training heavily. We knew how long of a walk I had and how long the ceremony would be, so I had clear goals.

The Sunday before the wedding we were at church, I told Megan that I didn't feel well. We went straight home so I could take a nap. I woke up four hours later with a raging fever. Megan went online, and came back and started poking around my stomach. I yelped in pain. She put some clothes on me and took me to the hospital. Sure enough, I had appendicitis.

As easy as it would have been to wonder, "What's next?" I calmly accepted the situation. I knew by now that everything happens for a reason.

Those couple of days in the hospital set me back physically. I told Megan I was afraid of walking down the aisle with her and making a big scene by tripping on her wedding dress or something. I didn't want to risk ruining our special day with me falling on my face. I did want to stand with her through the ceremony, though. I proposed that we do it the old-fashioned way, where I'd already be at the altar when she entered the chapel, and her dad would walk her down the aisle instead of me.

My son was my best man, and my best friend, Pete, was a groomsman. Megan's cousin, Malloree, was her maid of honor, and my daughter was a bridesmaid. A small crowd of friends and family gathered as Megan's father, Johnny, walked her down the aisle. I sat in anticipation. When the music started, I stood up as Megan and Johnny came down the isle. Then Megan took my hands as we stood before the pastor. When it was time, we exchanged vows, placed rings on our fingers, and enjoyed our first kiss as a married couple.

When our pastor announced us husband and wife, everyone cheered. Once again, there was a local news station there to film the ceremony.

Grinning, I lowered myself back onto my chair. Megan hopped onto my lap, and we sped down the aisle with me playfully swerving back and forth.

Of all the blessings and miracles that came after my accident, the most amazing one was Megan. Here was a young woman who had so many options in life, who could have done anything, and yet she chose to spend those critical years with me.

It's not being overdramatic or sentimental to say that I would not be here without her. I would have died in those first few nights if she hadn't been. Without her dedication and encouragement during rehab, I would not have wanted to continue living in the face of the pain and worry. My family would have fallen apart without her resilient demeanor, calm presence, and practical insight.

I'm overwhelmed with gratitude that she chose to sleep in that chair in the early days in the ICU. Later, she spent her nights on an uncomfortable cot in the rehab hospital. Even when we moved home, she slept on the couch next to my hospital bed. She never left my side even for one night of peaceful, uninterrupted sleep.

As time has passed, I have often found myself forgetting what brought me here. I've been in this chair for years. I've gotten used to being paralyzed as my life has fallen into a routine that isn't immune to the trials and tribulations of anyone else's life. The tendency is to get so caught up in "life" that I forget the gifts that God has given me.

It is at these times I think about how far I've come. How many people, including Megan, gave me their time, effort, resources, and, most of all, their love to inspire me to keep going. I refocus and retain a grateful mindset for the people and resources that have been placed in my path. "All I've wanted you to do was sing," He said. It is my mission to return all of that love by telling my story and passing that inspiration on to you.

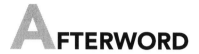

# AFTERWORD

This book was never going to be written. I had no interest in it. I was so focused on survival and making a living that I didn't take time to reflect on how awesome my recovery had been.

People ask me what happened. It is a natural response. They see a seemingly healthy guy in an electric wheelchair. Was it disease? An accident? When I tell them the whole story, they are astonished and almost unanimously have the same reaction, "You have to write a book."

As the years went by and I continued to recover incrementally, people would comment on my improvements. They would also ask, "What do they say is your prognosis?"

I first have to explain there is no "they" anymore. There is no doctor, nurse, or therapist who could predict what feeling and movement I would recover. I do know this, however, I have gotten back way more than "they" ever anticipated.

Nearly three years after the accident I found myself falling into my old patterns. I was taking things for granted, stressing about work, and putting my business life in front of my family again. Worse, I found that I had begun to forget the story and all the people and cool things that I had experienced.

One morning, I realized I had not been singing of Him, at least not to my full potential. Maybe I wasn't dancing like I used to, but work and routine had lulled me into forgetfulness about all that God had given me.

In the weeks and months after my accident, my very living and healing had been a testament to Him. He was healing me; He was giving me the strength to accomplish my audacious goals.

But now, people were used to me being in a wheelchair. The improvements, though continuing, were not as dramatic. And with my focus on work, I was neglecting my song.

I vowed that this could not continue. I needed to find a new way to sing, to reach out to more and more people. I needed new arenas where I could share my song. And I figured it would begin best with a book that could be read and shared.

I began to ask people if they knew anyone who could help me write a book. I didn't get much traction, certainly no referrals I wanted to work with.

One day, out of the blue, I received an email from Jonathan Peters, promoting the book of a client of his. Jonathan had been a colleague of mine before the accident, but we hadn't seen much of each other in the passing years. He was an English professor at UNLV, and, it turned out, he had ghostwritten dozens of books.

I called him, and we began the dialogue that resulted in this book. His first suggestion was that we begin by recording my story. I spent hours with a woman he recommended who would come over to my house and prompt me with questions. She would record me as I told my story. Simply reliving those stories with a person I hadn't known before the accident reminded me of all that I had accomplished and what God had done for me, that my story was worth telling, and that the lessons I had learned would have an impact on people's lives. What I wasn't prepared for is what a journey the process of creating this book would be. It changed my life again.

It is often said that God puts ordinary people in extraordinary circumstances. He put me in an extraordinary circumstance so I could share this message with you. The incredible journey that spurred me to write this book, forced me to "sing." By telling the whole story and what role God took in my recovery, I had to acknowledge my beliefs and my faith, which previously I had never done and I was always uncomfortable doing.

You go out on a limb when you talk about God and what He's done for you. Some of the people who are close to you are surprised, and may even judge you in ways you did not anticipate. Others will be delighted and welcome your confessions.

I had to be honest with myself and ask what I wanted to accomplish with my book. For those of faith, I hope that my "song" reaffirms your belief. I want you to be reminded that the power of prayer, combined with great attitude and effort, can make miracles happen. And I hope this book encourages you to sing your song of faith to others. It is the greatest gift you can give.

For those who are not of a certain faith or simply don't believe in God, I hope my experiences and realizations move you to find a relationship with a higher being. By yourself, you can overcome many things with a good attitude and great effort, but with a connection and a belief in a higher power, incredible, and even supernatural, things can happen. You owe it to yourself, your family, and your community to yield to the awesome power of God. Take it from a man who spent so much of his life dancing without Him, life with God is so much more rewarding and meaningful.

In the end, we have these days to explore and enjoy the gifts that are all around us. All of us face limitations and frustrations, some of us tragedies; it's the nature of life on this earth. But we have a choice of how we face difficulties, and more important, how we thrive, during them and afterwards. God's love helps us to thrive and magnifies each accomplishment as we overcome life's adversities.

Thank you for listening to my song.

Thank you for reading, and I sincerely hope you enjoyed, *Livin' on a Chair*. As an independently published author, I rely on you, the reader, to spread the word. So if you enjoyed the book, please tell your friends and family about it. And if it isn't too much trouble, I would appreciate a brief review on Amazon. If you are interested in booking me as a motivational speaker, please visit LivinOnaChair.com. Thanks again for your continued support.

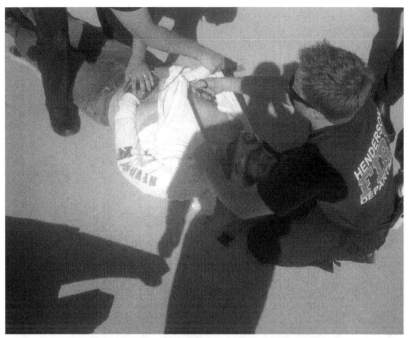

On the scene when Fire and Rescue arrived

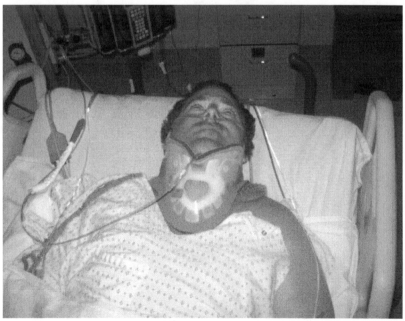

After surgery

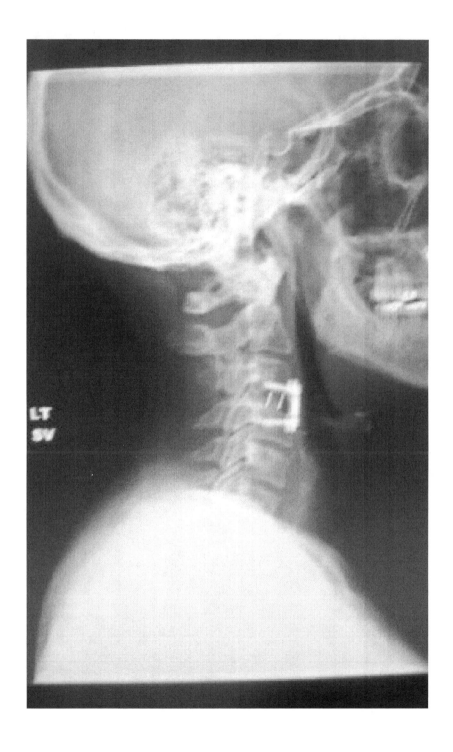

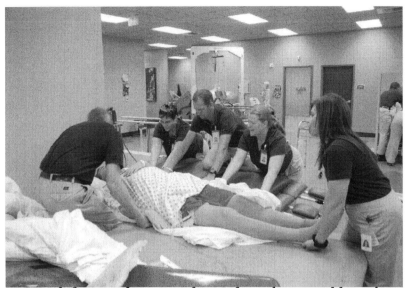

It took five people to transfer me from therapy table to the
gurney

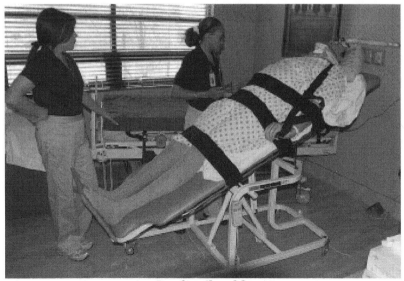

On the tilt table

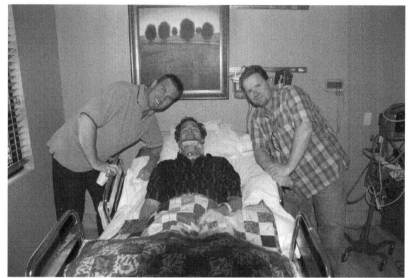

Cort Smith, me, and Ron Bishop

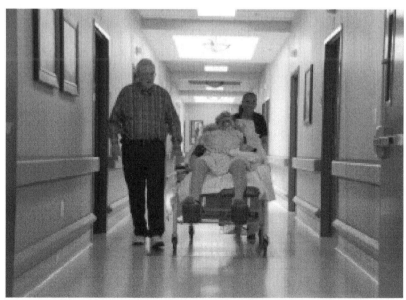

Rolling down the hall in my Cadillac chair with Dad

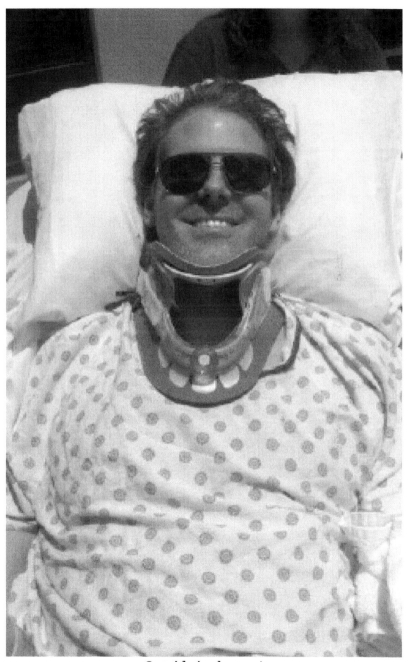

Outside in the sun!

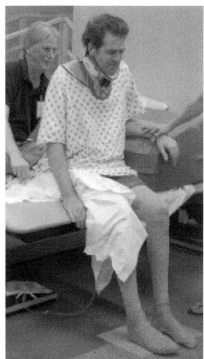

Sitting up, fighting nausea
and dropping blood pressure

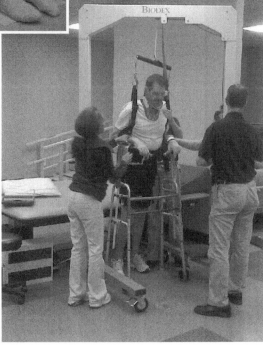

In the gait walker
with Ed and Deborah

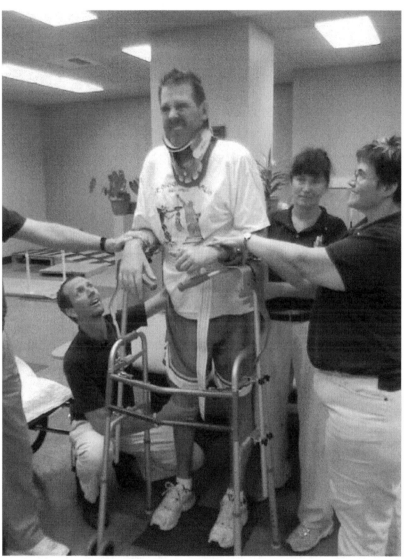

First step (note at the expression on everyone's faces)

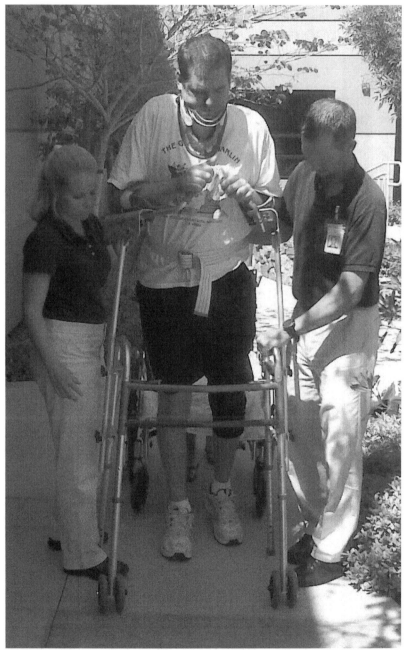

Using the platform walker outside

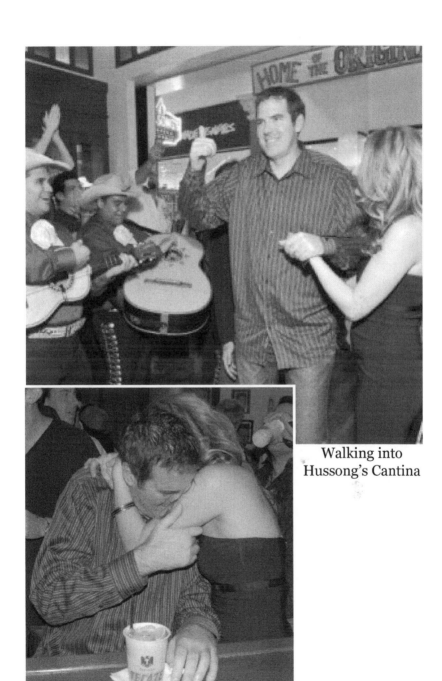

Walking into
Hussong's Cantina

Embracing after
the walk

213

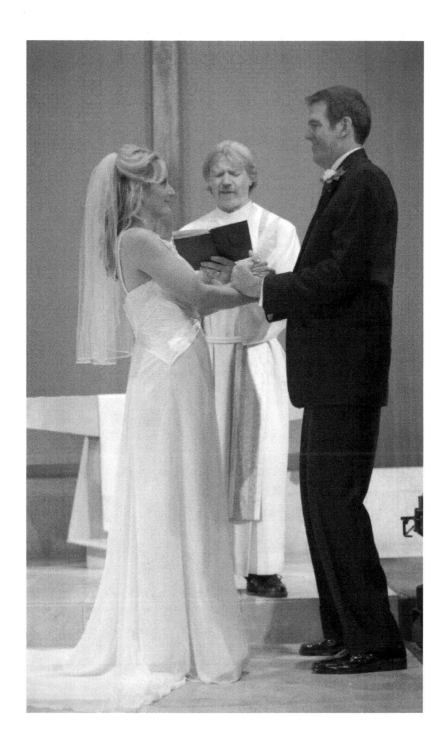

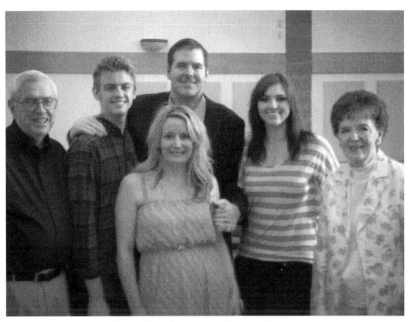
Family photo, August, 2013
From left to right: Ray (dad), Christian (son), Megan, Me,
Taylor (daughter), Gayle (mom)

The story continues on Facebook:
www.facebook.com/scottallenfrost

Please share your thoughts on twitter with #scottallenfrost

For newly paralyzed patients and their family and friends, please access the resources at the Spinal Injury Recovery Foundation at www.sirfus.org. We uploaded what we learned going through the process. Also, feel comfortable reaching out to us directly. We are here to support you.